Biomarkers for Heart Failure

Editor

TORU SUZUKI

HEART FAILURE CLINICS

www.heartfailure.theclinics.com

Consulting Editor
EDUARDO BOSSONE

Founding Editor
JAGAT NARULA

January 2018 • Volume 14 • Number 1

ELSEVIER

1600 John F. Kennedy Boulevard • Suite 1800 • Philadelphia, Pennsylvania, 19103-2899

http://www.theclinics.com

HEART FAILURE CLINICS Volume 14, Number 1
January 2018 ISSN 1551-7136, ISBN-13: 978-0-323-56641-4

Editor: Stacy Eastman
Developmental Editor: Laura Fisher

Heart Failure Clinics (ISSN 1551-7136) is published quarterly by Elsevier Inc., 360 Park Avenue South, New York, NY 10010-1710. Months of publication are January, April, July, and October. Business and editorial offices: 1600 John F. Kennedy Boulevard, Suite 1800, Philadelphia, PA 19103-2899. Periodicals postage paid at New York, NY, and additional mailing offices. Subscription prices are USD 252.00 per year for US individuals, USD 471.00 per year for US institutions, USD 100.00 per year for US students and residents, USD 294.00 per year for Canadian individuals, USD 545.00 per year for Canadian institutions, USD 309.00 per year for international individuals, USD 545.00 per year for international institutions, and USD 100.00 per year for Canadian and foreign students/residents. To receive student and resident rate, orders must be accompanied by name of affiliated institution, date of term, and the *signature* of program/residency coordinator on institution letterhead. Orders will be billed at individual rate until proof of status is received. Foreign air speed delivery is included in all *Clinics* subscription prices. All prices are subject to change without notice. **POSTMASTER:** Send address changes to *Heart Failure Clinics*, Elsevier Health Sciences Division, Subscription Customer Service, 3251 Riverport Lane, Maryland Heights, MO 63043. **Customer Service: 1-800-654-2452 (US and Canada). From outside of the US and Canada, call 314-447-8871. Fax: 314-447-8029. For print support, E-mail: JournalsCustomerService-usa@elsevier.com. For online support, E-mail: JournalsOnlineSupport-usa@elsevier.com.**

Reprints. For copies of 100 or more of articles in this publication, please contact the Commercial Reprints Department, Elsevier Inc., 360 Park Avenue South, New York, NY 10010-1710. Tel.: 212-633-3874; Fax: 212-633-3820; E-mail: reprints@elsevier.com.

Heart Failure Clinics is covered in *MEDLINE/PubMed (Index Medicus).*

Contributors

CONSULTING EDITOR

EDUARDO BOSSONE, MD, PhD, FESC, FACC
'Cava de' Tirreni and Amalfi Coast,' Division of Cardiology, Heart Department, University Hospital, Salerno, Italy

EDITOR

TORU SUZUKI, MD, PhD
Professor, Cardiovascular Medicine, Department of Cardiovascular Sciences, NIHR Biomedical Research Centre, University of Leicester, Glenfield Hospital, Leicester, United Kingdom; Jichi Medical University, Tochigi-ken, Japan

AUTHORS

CHONYANG L. ALBERT, MD
Department of Cardiovascular Medicine, Heart & Vascular Institute, Cleveland Clinic, Cleveland, Ohio, USA

MICHELE ARCOPINTO, MD
Department of Translational Medical Sciences, Federico II University, Naples, Italy

EMANUELE BOBBIO, MD
Department of Translational Medical Sciences, Federico II University, Naples, Italy

EDUARDO BOSSONE, MD, PhD, FESC, FACC
'Cava de' Tirreni and Amalfi Coast,' Division of Cardiology, Heart Department, University Hospital, Salerno, Italy

THONG HUY CAO, MD, PhD
Postdoctoral Research Associate, Department of Cardiovascular Sciences, NIHR Biomedical Research Centre, University of Leicester, Glenfield Hospital, Leicester, United Kingdom; Lecturer and Cardiologist, Department of General Internal Medicine, University of Medicine and Pharmacy, Ho Chi Minh City, Vietnam

ANTONIO CITTADINI, MD
Department of Translational Medical Sciences, Federico II University, Interdisciplinary Research Centre in Biomedical Materials (CRIB), Naples, Italy

ROBERTA D'ASSANTE, PhD
IRCCS SDN, Naples, Italy

RUDOLF A. DE BOER, MD, PhD, FESC, FHFA
Department of Cardiology, University of Groningen, University Medical Center Groningen, Groningen, The Netherlands

JASON M. DURAN, MD, PhD
Department of Internal Medicine, UC San Diego, San Diego, California, USA

GREGG C. FONAROW, MD
Professor, Division of Cardiology, Department of Medicine, Ronald Reagan UCLA Medical Center, Los Angeles, California, USA

CAROLIN GEHLKEN, MD
Department of Cardiology, University of Groningen, University Medical Center Groningen, Groningen, The Netherlands

LIAM M. HEANEY, PhD
Department of Cardiovascular Sciences, NIHR
Biomedical Research Centre, University of
Leicester, Glenfield Hospital, Leicester, United
Kingdom

MUHAMMAD ZUBAIR ISRAR, MSc
Department of Cardiovascular Sciences, NIHR
Biomedical Research Centre, University of
Leicester, Glenfield Hospital, Leicester, United
Kingdom

JAMES L. JANUZZI Jr, MD, FACC
Division of Cardiology, Department of
Medicine, Massachusetts General Hospital,
Baim Institute for Clinical Research,
Cardiometabolic Trials, Boston,
Massachusetts, USA

ALAN S. MAISEL, MD, FACC
Professor of Medicine, Division of Cardiology,
UC San Diego, Division of Cardiovascular
Medicine, VA San Diego Healthcare System,
San Diego, California, USA

ALBERTO M. MARRA, MD
IRCCS SDN, Naples, Italy

CIAN P. McCARTHY, MB, BCh, BAO
Department of Medicine, Massachusetts
General Hospital, Boston, Massachusetts,
USA

WOUTER C. MEIJERS, MD, PhD, FHFA
Department of Cardiology, University of
Groningen, University Medical Center
Groningen, Groningen, The Netherlands

YASUAKI NAKAGAWA, MD, PhD
Assistant Professor, Department of
Cardiovascular Medicine, Graduate School of
Medicine Kyoto University, Kyoto, Japan

LEONG LOKE NG, MA, MD
Professor of Medicine and Therapeutics,
Department of Cardiovascular Sciences, NIHR
Biomedical Research Centre, University of
Leicester, Glenfield Hospital, Leicester, United
Kingdom

TOSHIO NISHIKIMI, MD, PhD
Clinical Professor, Department of
Cardiovascular Medicine, Graduate School of
Medicine Kyoto University, Kyoto, Japan;
Director, Department of Medicine, Wakakusa
Tatsuma Rehabilitation Hospital, Daito City,
Osaka, Japan

**ARTHUR MARK RICHARDS, MBChB, MD,
PhD, DSc**
Director, Cardiovascular Research Institute,
National University of Singapore, National
University Heart Centre, Singapore, Singapore;
Director, Christchurch Heart Institute,
University of Otago, Christchurch, New
Zealand

ANDREA SALZANO, MD
Department of Translational Medical Sciences,
Federico II University, Naples, Italy;
Department of Cardiovascular Sciences, NIHR
Biomedical Research Centre, University of
Leicester, Glenfield Hospital, Leicester, United
Kingdom

KEVIN S. SHAH, MD
Fellow of Cardiovascular Disease, University of
California, Los Angeles, Los Angeles,
California, USA

**DANIEL CHU SIONG CHAN, BMedSci,
BMBS**
Clinical Research Fellow, Department of
Cardiovascular Sciences, NIHR Biomedical
Research Centre, University of Leicester,
Glenfield Hospital, Leicester,
United Kingdom

NAVIN SUTHAHAR, MD
Department of Cardiology, University of
Groningen, University Medical Center
Groningen, Groningen, The Netherlands

TORU SUZUKI, MD, PhD
Professor, Cardiovascular Medicine,
Department of Cardiovascular Sciences, NIHR
Biomedical Research Centre, University of
Leicester, Glenfield Hospital, Leicester, United
Kingdom; Jichi Medical University, Tochigi-
ken, Japan

W.H. WILSON TANG, MD
Department of Cardiovascular Medicine, Heart
& Vascular Institute, Center for Clinical
Genomics, Cleveland Clinic, Cleveland, Ohio,
USA

NICHOLAS WETTERSTEN, MD
Division of Cardiovascular Medicine, UC San
Diego, San Diego, California, USA

Contents

> The opioid system is activated in heart failure, which may be cardioprotective but also may be counterregulatory. Recently, systemic proenkephalin activation has been investigated in various conditions predicting mortality and kidney injury. In acute heart failure, proenkephalin independently predicts mortality and heart failure rehospitalization in addition to traditional risk markers. It also predicts worsening renal function, increasingly recognized as an important risk predictor for poor outcome in heart failure. This article explores the role of enkephalins and delta-opioid receptors in the heart, then reviews studies measuring proenkephalin levels in the circulation and their associations with prognosis.

> The natriuretic peptides play a vital role in normal physiology and as counterregulatory hormones in heart failure (HF). Clinical assessment of their levels (for B-type natriuretic peptide [BNP], N-terminal proBNP, and the midregion of N-terminal pro–atrial natriuretic peptide) have become valuable tools in diagnosing patients with HF as well as risk stratifying and guiding therapy. Their roles have further expanded beyond HF to other cardiovascular conditions and for risk stratification in asymptomatic individuals. Understanding the clinical use of these hormones is vital to achieving their full potential.

> Plasma amino-terminal pro–B-type natriuretic peptide (NT-proBNP) is a guideline-mandated biomarker in heart failure (HF). Used as an inclusion criterion for therapeutic trials, NT-proBNP enriches trial populations and is a valid surrogate endpoint. Its diagnostic performance is best validated in acute decompensated HF (ADHF). NT-proBNP offers prognostic information independent of standard clinical predictors and refines risk stratification. With the advent of combined angiotensin 2 type 1 receptor blockade and neprilysin inhibition (ARNI), NT-proBNP retains its relationship to cardiac status and is the marker of choice in assessment of possible ADHF and in serial monitoring of HF patients receiving ARNI treatment.

> Suppression of tumorigenicity 2 (ST2) is a member of the interleukin (IL)-1 receptor family, whose role was originally established in the context of inflammatory and autoimmune diseases. More recently, testing for ST2 has been used in the setting of cardiovascular disease. The soluble form of ST2 is a decoy receptor that inhibits

beneficial cardioprotective effects of IL-33; such inhibition results in cardiac hypertrophy, myocardial fibrosis, and ventricular dysfunction. Measurement of soluble ST2 has utility for assessing heart failure severity and prognosis. In this review, we examine the role of soluble ST2 in both acute and chronic heart failure.

Adrenomedullin (AM) is a vasodilatory peptide originally discovered in human pheochromocytoma tissue. Although AM is highly expressed in the adrenal glands, heart, lungs, and kidneys, vascular endothelium and smooth muscle are thought to be the main source of plasma AM. The AM precursor is processed to AM-glycine, which is then converted to AM-mature through C-terminal amidation. In this process, mid-regional pro-adrenomedullin (MR-proAM) is also produced. Plasma AM, AM-mature, AM-glycine, and MR-proAM levels are all higher in patients with heart failure than healthy subjects in proportion to the disease severity. All molecular forms of AM are prognostic markers for heart failure.

Cardiac troponin is an integral biomarker in the evaluation and management of patients with acute coronary syndrome. Troponin is also established as a valuable prognostic marker in patients with acute or chronic heart failure (HF). As the sensitivity of troponin assays transition to high sensitive troponin, more patients with HF will have detectable troponin. In this review, the authors discuss the current literature on the value of troponin in the management of patients with HF. Furthermore, the authors highlight the potential for future strategies to use troponin as a potential target for therapy in patients with HF.

The impairment of growth hormone (GH)/insulin growth factor-1(IGF-1) plays a crucial role in chronic heart failure (CHF). Several studies have shown that patients affected by this condition display a more aggressive disease, with impaired functional capacity and poor outcomes. Interestingly, GH replacement therapy represents a possible future therapeutic option in CHF. In this article, the authors focus on the assessment of the main abnormalities in GH/IGF-1 axis in CHF, the underlying molecular background, and their impact on disease progression and outcomes.

Galectin-3 plays a role in tissue inflammation, repair, and fibrosis. This article specifically focuses on heart failure (HF), in which galectin-3 has been shown to be a useful biomarker in prognosis and risk stratification, especially in HF with preserved ejection fraction. Experimental research has shown that galectin-3 directly induces pathologic remodeling of the heart, and is therefore considered a culprit protein in the development of cardiac fibrosis in HF, with potentially relevant clinical implications. In summary, galectin-3 is a biomarker and biotarget in cardiac remodeling and fibrosis and future research will target galectin-3–centered diseases.

Heart failure (HF) is associated with significant morbidity and mortality. Biomarkers are used to assist clinicians with timely diagnosis, prognosis, and risk prediction of patients for personalized treatment. Using modern proteomic methods such as mass spectrometry, an increasing number of novel biomarkers have been identified that further aid clinicians in the early diagnosis and outcome prediction of HF. This article focuses on the array of common and novel protein-based biomarkers that provide diagnostic and prognostic information in HF.

Metabolomics is the study of small, organic molecules within biochemical pathways. With advancement of technology, nuclear magnetic resonance, gas chromatography, and mass spectrometry have allowed for the discovery and analysis of large databases of metabolites implicated in heart failure. Metabolomics also explores the patient and environmental interactions and unlocks the link between environmental exposures and the development of cardiovascular disease. Although a relatively new field, metabolomics is poised to become a clinically impactful field that develops novel biomarkers and explores new therapeutic interventions in heart failure.

HEART FAILURE CLINICS

THE CLINICS ARE AVAILABLE ONLINE!
Access your subscription at:
www.theclinics.com

Preface
Biomarkers of Heart Failure: Past, Present, and Future

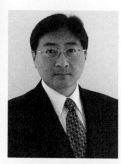
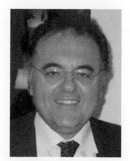

Toru Suzuki, MD, PhD
Editor

Eduardo Bossone, MD, PhD, FESC, FACC
Consulting Editor

Biomarkers are used in routine patient care to diagnose, monitor (response to treatment), and risk stratify/prognosticate patients with heart failure. The "golden standard" biomarker that is currently used clinically is arguably B-type natriuretic peptide (BNP), yet it has still only been a little over a quarter century ago that the natriuretic peptides were identified and were clinically translated for use in the diagnosis of heart failure years after the initial discovery.[1,2] Time flies fast. Junior doctors of today would surely not be able to even imagine a time when we didn't have such "tool(s)" available at the bedside. When BNP was initially investigated, heart failure only referred to what we now know to be that with reduced ejection fraction. There is now heart failure with preserved ejection fraction, and we are also now better able to define an intermediary "remodeling" process with the contribution of advanced imaging methods to better define pathologies in a noninvasive manner. With global aging and contribution of better health/heart care, there is a demographic landscape for heart failure that is ever changing. On top of that, there are expectations that medicine will be done in a "precise" manner (precision medicine), meaning that we will go beyond the simplified binary diagnostic models of yesteryear to produce real-time personalized assessments based on multifaceted clinical and biological data (eg, multi-omics approaches). Perhaps artificial intelligence-assisted medicine will become the norm to process the multitude of information. Biomarkers reflecting different pathologies and approaches ("omics") need to be investigated, including refinements and new discoveries. Nobody knows what the future will hold, but one thing that is clear is that our patient care at present is defined by past discoveries, and that future medicine will be predicated by discoveries of today.[3] This issue provides up-to-date knowledge on contemporary achievements and discoveries that may be further translated to patient care. In closing, we would like to thank all of the contributing authors for their time in preparing their sections for this issue.

Toru Suzuki, MD, PhD
Department of Cardiovascular Sciences
University of Leicester
Glenfield Hospital
Groby Road
Leicester LE3 9QP, United Kingdom

Eduardo Bossone, MD, PhD, FESC, FACC
'Cava de' Tirreni and Amalfi Coast'
Division of Cardiology
Heart Department
University Hospital
Salerno, Italy

E-mail addresses:
ts263@le.ac.uk (T. Suzuki)
ebossone@hotmail.com (E. Bossone)

Heart Failure Clin 14 (2018) ix–x
http://dx.doi.org/10.1016/j.hfc.2017.08.012
1551-7136/18/© 2017 Published by Elsevier Inc.

REFERENCES

1. Suzuki T, Yamaki Y, Yazaki Y. The role of the natriuretic peptides in the cardiovascular system. Cardiovasc Res 2001;3:489–94.
2. Suzuki T. Cardiovascular diagnostic biomarkers: the past, present and future. Circ J 2009;73:806–9.
3. Suzuki T, Nagai R. Molecular markers for cardiovascular disease: cardiovascular biomarkers to proteomic discovery. Nat Clin Pract Cardiovasc Med 2008; 5:295.

Proenkephalin in Heart Failure

Daniel Chu Siong Chan, BMedSci, BMBS[a,1], Thong Huy Cao, MD, PhD[a,b,1],
Leong Loke Ng, MA, MD[a,*]

KEYWORDS

• Proenkephalin • PENK • Heart failure • Delta-opioid receptor • Enkephalin • Renal function

KEY POINTS

- The endogenous opioid system plays an important role in cardioprotection and is activated in heart failure.
- Proenkephalin is a precursor for endogenous enkephalins, which in turn activate delta-opioid receptors in various tissues.
- In the heart, delta-opioid receptor activation results in reduced myocardial contractility, blood pressure, and heart rate, but in kidneys it increases renal blood flow and urine output.
- Circulating Proenkephalin-A (PENK), a surrogate for enkephalin synthesis from proenkephalin, predicts poor outcomes in myocardial infarction and heart failure, and with additional predictive value.
- Adding PENK to a decision-making process helps physicians predict risk more accurately, and could improve treatment selection in these patients.

BACKGROUND

The opioid system has been well studied and characterized in the nervous system, but interest has been mounting in its importance in the cardiovascular system.[1] Endogenous opioid peptides, which interact with receptors for morphine, subsequently named enkephalins, were first reported by Kosterlitz and Hughes[2] in 1975. Besides Met-enkephalin and Leu-enkephalin, several other enkephalin-containing peptides have been discovered, all of which have varying degrees of specificity on opioid receptors. Although enkephalins were first characterized in brain and adrenal glands through the use of immunohistochemistry,[3] both enkephalins and opioid receptors have since been identified in the central nervous system in the adrenal medulla, dorsal vagus nucleus, nucleus ambiguus, nucleus tractus solitarius, and in the peripheral nervous system in sympathetic and parasympathetic neurones of the heart, spleen, vas deferens, stomach, intestine, lung, pancreas, and liver.[4,5]

Opioid peptides arise from pro-opiomelanocortin, prodynorphin, and proenkephalin, the precursors for endorphins, dynorphins, and enkephalins respectively. These peptides are the endogenous ligands for the 3 types of opioid receptors: µ-opioid receptors, κ-opioid receptors, and δ-opioid receptors respectively.[6,7] These peptides have been found to affect various physiologic activities, including respiration, sleep, immune function, endocrine function, body temperature, attention, catatonia, and drug dependence.[8–12]

The opioid system also plays an important role in the cardiovascular system, for which evidence

Disclosure: T.H. Cao is funded by the John and Lucille van Geest Foundation. D.C.S. Chan is funded by the British Heart Foundation on grant FS/15/10/31223. L.L. Ng has nothing to disclose.
[a] Department of Cardiovascular Sciences, NIHR Biomedical Research Centre, University of Leicester, Glenfield Hospital, Groby Road, Leicester LE3 9QP, UK; [b] Department of General Internal Medicine, University of Medicine and Pharmacy, Hong Bang Street, Ward 11, District 5, Ho Chi Minh City, Vietnam
[1] These two authors contributed equally.
* Corresponding author.
E-mail address: lln1@leicester.ac.uk

heartfailure.theclinics.com

has been accumulating over the past 3 decades. These regulatory roles occur at both the central and peripheral levels. Activation of opioid peptide receptors by their respective endogenous ligands results in different effects on heart rate and blood pressure, depending on the animal species, agonist route, administration, and anesthetic use.[13–15] In general, opioid peptide receptor stimulation causes hypotension and bradycardia. However, activation of δ-opioid receptors in the nucleus tractus solitarius or cisterna causes hypertension and tachycardia, whereas activation of the κ-opioid receptors in the same place causes biphasic effects on blood pressure.

In light of recent work on the emerging role of proenkephalin as a marker for prognosis, this article first focuses on the relevance of enkephalin and its precursor proenkephalin in the cardiovascular system, followed by an overview of the emerging evidence for proenkephalin's role in prognosis in heart failure.

ENKEPHALINS IN THE HEART

Although enkephalins are produced and released in the central nervous system and in peripheral neuronal terminals in the heart, where they are coreleased with catecholamines,[4] most enkephalins produced in the heart are from cardiomyocytes.[16,17] Enkephalins are synthesized from preproenkephalin A, which has 267 amino acids.[18,19] Cleavage of the N-terminal signal sequence gives rise to proenkephalin (243 amino acids),[20] which subsequently undergoes further posttranslational processing to produce 4 Met-enkephalins, 1 Leu-enkephalin, the heptapeptide Met-enkephalin-Arg-Phe and the octapeptide Met-enkephalin-Arg-Gly-Lys, as well as other analogues and intermediates (**Fig. 1**). Proenkephalin messenger RNA (mRNA) has been shown to be higher in heart than brain; however, smaller quantities of mature enkephalin peptides can be extracted from the heart.[21,22] Most of the enkephalin-containing peptides recovered from rat ventricle are concentrated in larger-molecular-weight intermediary peptides,[23] which could provide a ready source for the myocardium to use to synthesize mature enkephalins in times of need.[24] Posttranslational processing of proenkephalin is tissue specific,[25] resulting in different intermediates. After synthesis, circulating enkephalins are rapidly degraded by neutral endopeptidases (also known as enkephalinases),[26,27] giving them a half-life of less than 15 minutes.[28] These membrane-bound endopeptidases are present in cardiomyocytes,[29] implying that enkephalins have an autocrine/paracrine effect, being produced and degraded locally as required. However, there are other sites of high enkephalinase activity, such as the kidneys and lungs,[30] which could remove circulating enkephalins.

CARDIOPROTECTION

Enkephalins have been found to play a role in ischemic preconditioning. Ischemic preconditioning describes the protection from ischemic events following episodes of brief sublethal ischemia,[31] which reduces myocardial infarct size and improves functional recovery. Animal studies with specific opioid peptide receptor antagonism

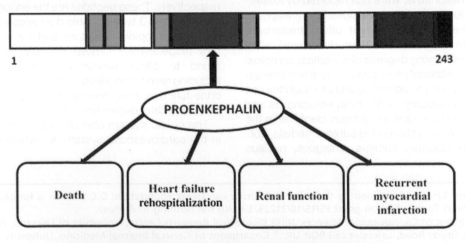

(Green: Met-Enk, Red: Proenkephalin: 119–159, Blue: Met-Enk-RGL, Yellow: Leu-Enk, Purple: Enkelytin, Navy: Met-Enk-RF.)

Fig. 1. Role of proenkephalin in prognosis for patients with cardiovascular diseases. Leu-Enk, Leu-enkephalin; Met-Enk, Met-enkephalin; Met-Enk-RF, Met-enkephalin Arginine Phenylalanine; Met-Enk-RGL, Met-enkephalin Arginine glycine leucine.

show that ischemic preconditioning depends on δ-opioid receptors but not μ-opioid receptors or κ-opioid receptors.[32,33] Endurance exercise promotes cardiac protection against myocardial ischemia-reperfusion injury, also through a δ-opioid receptor–dependent process, involving downregulation of δ-opioid receptor and κ-opioid receptor.[34] Nevertheless, the downstream mechanisms that underpin this cardioprotection are not fully understood, although most evidence implicates cardiac mitochondria,[35] where mitochondrial ATP-sensitive potassium channels open to prevent cytosolic calcium overload.[36] Activation of δ-opioid receptor and κ-opioid receptor protects cardiomyocytes via mitochondrial potassium-ATP channels.[37] In addition, opioid peptide receptor inhibition by naloxone abolishes the cardiac protection offered by ischemic preconditioning.[38,39] Parallels can be drawn from nature regarding the potential evolutionary benefit for ischemic preconditioning. Hibernation in cold-weather and ischemic preconditioning share a similar process, both of which can be abolished by δ-opioid receptor inhibition.[40] Further evidence for its relevance comes from gene expression profiling of human hibernating myocardium, which found increased expression of proenkephalin in these tissues compared with normally contracting regions.[41]

REGULATION OF CELLULAR LIFE CYCLE

Enkephalins participate in growth through a different receptor known as the opioid growth factor receptor (OGFr), previously known as the zeta (ζ) opioid receptor. The specific endogenous ligand for this receptor is Met5-enkephalin, one of 4 Met-enkephalins synthesized from proenkephalin. These receptors have been shown to be distinct from classic opioid receptors. OGFr activation inhibits normal cell and cancer cell proliferation by inhibiting the G_0/S phases of the cell cycle. The OGFr protein and gene expression have a wide distribution akin to that of enkephalins, of neural and nonneural origin, and have been detected in mouse brain, heart, kidney, liver, and muscle.[42–44] Much like preproenkephalin, expression levels of the OGFr decline in adult tissues and nonreplicative organs.[44–46] This opioid growth factor (OGF)–OGFr axis tonically maintains homeostasis of proliferating cells and tissues and requires a change in balance of both components to change cell number. An increase in OGF or OGFr may inhibit cellular proliferation but the converse may be required in cases of wound healing or tissue repair. RNA sequencing of normal human tissues identified that OGFr expression is highest in spleen/lymphoid tissue with average

expression in kidney but one of the lowest in heart.[47] In addition to suppressing cellular proliferation, proenkephalin facilitates stress-activated apoptosis, a function thought to be caused by physical association of endogenous proenkephalin with the transcriptional corepressor histone deacetylase, following activation of nuclear factor κ-B or p53 pathways.[48] Although this alludes to the importance that opioids play in cellular proliferation both in physiologic and pathophysiologic states, with particular importance in tumorigenesis, whether or not enkephalins significantly regulate cellular proliferation in adult hearts (thought to be postmitotic) is unclear and warrants further investigation.

ENKEPHALINS IN HEART FAILURE

The role of the enkephalins in heart failure is not well characterized and probably complex with activation of the cardiac opioid system in congestive heart failure observed in animals.[49] In dogs, increased endogenous opioid levels during heart failure act on the δ-opioid receptors causing a decrease of myocardial mechanical performance and altering regional blood flow distribution.[50] Deranged intracellular calcium signaling and homeostasis have been implicated in heart failure.[51,52] Suppression of the L-type Ca^{2+}-current has been observed in response to enkephalin, resulting in reduced myocardial contractility[53] and δ-opioid receptor activation reduces the responsiveness of myofilaments to Ca^{2+}.[54] These opioid receptors are found to colocalize with the L-type Ca^{2+}-channel and the intracellular ryanodine receptor (RyR). In addition, both proenkephalin and δ-opioid receptor mRNA and their respective proteins were found to be upregulated in the left ventricle in heart failure.[55] Heart failure results in systemic sympathetic activation, and there seems to be some dependence of the opioid system on sympathetic activity. In isolated rat hearts, δ-opioid receptor inhibition resulted in increased blood pressure and cardiac contractility, but blockade of adrenergic beta-receptors abolished this effect. This finding could be caused by downstream cross-talk between beta-adrenergic sympathetic signaling and opioid receptor signaling.[56] β-Endorphin levels are increased in the ventricles of failing hearts,[49] and although the δ-opioid receptor is generally accepted to be principally responsible for regulating the vasopressor/depressor response of opioid peptides in heart failure, the μ-opioid receptor is thought to be responsible for the blunting of baroreceptor sensitivity in heart failure.[57]

In humans, β-endorphin levels have been found to be increased in congestive heart failure compared with healthy subjects and these increases were correlated with the patients' New York Heart Association functional cardiac status (control, 14.0 ± 4.4 pg/mL; class II, 17.9 ± 3.6 pg/mL; class III, 28.3 ± 8.8 pg/mL; class IV, 46.7 ± 14.6 pg/mL, mean ± SD).[58] In addition, in acute heart failure, atrial natriuretic factor (ANF), a neurohormone that causes diuresis and natriuresis, and correlates with the severity of heart failure, is also positively correlated with circulating opioid peptides (β-endorphin, dynorphin, and met-enkephalin). Nonspecific opioid receptor inhibition with naloxone significantly increased ANF levels, noradrenaline levels, heart rate, and blood pressure in severe heart failure, but, in less severe heart failure, naloxone decreased ANF levels, without change to noradrenaline, blood pressure, and heart rate.[59] The investigators hypothesized that this could be caused by sympathetic activity–dependent upregulation of the opioid system in heart failure, whereas more severe heart failure results in increased sympathetic activation.

Clinically, morphine is often used for rapid relief of respiratory distress in acute heart failure. Historically this was thought to occur through a reduction in ventricular preload, reducing work to the ventricles while other therapies, such as diuretics, take effect. Physiologic increases in β-endorphin levels support this notion, although the survival advantage of decreasing systemic blood pressure and heart rate as a result of opioid receptor activation is not immediately clear. Peacock and colleagues[60] performed a retrospective analysis of the Acute Decompensated Heart Failure National Registry (ADHERE), investigating whether there was a link between morphine administration in acute heart failure and mortality risk. Patients receiving morphine had more severe heart failure symptoms with rest dyspnea, more radiographic evidence of pulmonary congestion, and increased troponin levels. Morphine administration was associated with a higher risk of mechanical ventilation, intensive care unit admissions, and increased mortality. Mortality risk remained even after exclusion of ventilated patients and adjustment with odds ratio (OR) of 4.84 (95% confidence interval [CI], 4.52–5.18).

MEASURING PROENKEPHALIN

Ascertaining the activity of the enkephalin system has previously been difficult to perform and interpret, because of the short half-life of active enkephalins and the large number of intermediate peptides, some of which are of large molecular weight and unlikely to be released into the circulation until they have been postprocessed into active enkephalins. Human preproenkephalin A comprises 267 amino

acids and is widely distributed in the nervous system, adrenal medulla, bone-derived cells, and cells of the immune system. The N-terminal signal peptide is removed by a specific signal peptidase,[20] giving rise to a 243-amino-acid proenkephalin-A precursor protein (now named proenkephalin). This precursor can then be targeted by specific membrane-bound carboxypeptidases, also known as enkephalin convertases,[61] which cleave the C-terminal basic residues to form mature Met-enkephalin and Leu-enkephalin. Initially identified in adrenal chromaffin cells, they have also been measured in brain, with colocalization in areas where opioid receptors are most dense. They probably explain the tissue-specific nature of proenkephalin posttranslational processing that has been observed.[25,62–64] In addition to mature enkephalins, other peptides are produced, one of which is a stable proenkephalin peptide 119-159. This fragment is stable in plasma and cerebrospinal fluid for at least 48 hours at room temperature, and it this molecule for which a novel sandwich immunoassay has been developed (PENK).[65] This peptide fragment's levels in plasma/serum could serve as a surrogate measurement of systemic enkephalin synthesis, because proenkephalin is the predominant source of mature enkephalins. For the remainder of this article, PENK refers to the measurement of proenkephalin 119-159 using this assay, and proenkephalin refers to the precursor of mature enkephalins that has not been processed intracellularly.

PROENKEPHALIN IS A PROGNOSTIC MARKER IN SEVERAL DISEASES

Plasma PENK levels have been measured in a variety of prospective cohorts. In cerebrospinal fluid, PENK was strongly positively correlated with N-protachykinin A, a surrogate for substance P. Substance P is one of several signaling molecules released in response to nociception and is both a neurotransmitter and a neuromodulator[66,67] but has a plethora of other effects. Its levels are lower in both dementia and acute cerebral inflammation compared with healthy individuals.[68] In a prospective cohort of patients undergoing routine cardiac surgery, PENK predicts acute kidney injury, with a similar predictive capability to baseline creatinine.[69] In addition, in patients admitted to the emergency department for sepsis, PENK predicts acute kidney injury.[70] A recent study evaluated the prognostic value of PENK levels in 1141 patients with acute myocardial infarction by using N-terminal pro–B-type natriuretic peptide (NT-proBNP) and Global Registry of Acute Coronary Events (GRACE) scores as comparators. End points included major adverse events (composite of death, myocardial infarction, and heart failure hospitalization) and recurrent acute myocardial infarction at 2 years. The results showed that PENK levels reflected cardiorenal status after acute myocardial infarction and had a role as a predictor of major adverse events such as death, recurrent acute myocardial infarction, and heart failure. Cutoff values of PENK levels less than 48.3 pmol/L and greater than 91 pmol/L were able to define low-risk and high-risk patients and improve risk prediction of GRACE scores. The major determinant of PENK levels was renal function, and there was a strong negative correlation between PENK and estimated glomerular filtration rate (eGFR).[71] Furthermore, in healthy individuals, higher PENK level predicts the development of kidney disease in later life, and is positively associated with creatinine and cystatin C and negatively associated with eGFR.[72] In addition, Schulz and colleagues[72] identified a single nucleotide polymorphism on the locus encoding proenkephalin, which was associated with increased PENK levels and predicting kidney disease, implying potential causality of proenkephalin in the development of future kidney disease, although in-depth exploration is required.

Other examples of PENK predicting poor outcome are found in ischemic stroke, in which higher PENK level was related to stroke severity, functional disability, and mortality.[73] Plasma creatinine level was not a determinant of PENK levels. The investigators attribute the relation of PENK to prognosis with it being a marker of blood-brain barrier integrity, allowing the high levels of PENK in cerebrospinal fluid (100-fold higher than plasma[65]) to leak into the circulation. At present, it is not clear where most of the circulating plasma PENK is from, although Denning and colleagues[74] showed that multiple nonneuronal tissues express pre-proenkephalin mRNA, enkephalins, and associated δ-opioid receptors but they are of highest density in the kidney. In addition, lower PENK levels have been found to predict the development of breast cancer.[75] Markers of renal function were not reported in that publication; however, PENK levels measured in that study could be in keeping with the OGF-OGFr axis hypotheses. In a diabetic cohort, PENK did not predict long-term mortality. However, like other studies, it found a significant association of PENK with serum creatinine.[76] **Table 1** summarizes the non–heart failure studies that have used PENK to provide prognostic information.

PROENKEPHALIN IN HEART FAILURE

There have been very few studies so far that evaluate the role of PENK in cardiovascular diseases, especially in heart failure. Several main studies and roles of proenkephalin in cardiovascular diseases are described later.

PROENKEPHALIN IS A MARKER FOR RISK STRATIFICATION IN STABLE MINIMALLY SYMPTOMATIC OR ASYMPTOMATIC AMBULATORY COMMUNITY-DWELLING PATIENTS

PENK may have a useful role in classifying risk for stable patients with heart failure. Arbit and colleagues[77] performed the first study to evaluate the prognostic role of PENK in stable ambulatory patients. Two-hundred patients with American College of Cardiology (ACC)/American Heart Association (AHA) stages A and B heart failure were recruited in a 4-year prospective cohort study. The end points of cardiovascular-related hospital admission or death were assessed. PENK levels were higher in patients who had a higher serum creatinine level and lower eGFR, lower left ventricular ejection fraction (LVEF), hypertension, and diabetes. After 3.5 years of follow-up, the highest PENK tertile had a hazard ratio of 3.0 (95% CI, 1.4–6.7) compared with the lowest tertile ($P<.007$) for the primary end point. However, this study had its limitations, having been conducted in a single center with 98% of patients being male, and only patients with ACC/AHA stages A and B were included in the analysis.[77]

PROENKEPHALIN IS A MARKER OF PROGNOSIS IN PATIENTS WITH HEART FAILURE

In light of the strong associations between PENK and renal function, Matsue and colleagues[78] investigated, in a cohort of patients with chronic heart failure, the association between PENK, glomerular function, and tubular function. PENK was strongly associated with glomerular function but not tubular function. The investigators also studied the link between PENK and clinical outcomes in 1589 patients with acute heart failure who fulfilled the inclusion criteria for a drug trial (rolofylline). PENK levels were higher in patients with both acute and chronic heart failure compared with normal subjects. Furthermore, PENK level was higher in acute heart failure compared with chronic heart failure. In the acute heart failure group, PENK was able to predict death at 180 days, heart failure rehospitalization at 60 days, and death or cardiovascular or renal rehospitalization at day 60 in univariable analyses, but its predictive value was lost in a multivariable model when adjustments to the

Table 1
Summary of non–heart failure studies using PENK to provide prognostic information

Author	Type of Study	Number of Patients	Inclusion Criteria	End Points	HR, OR, or AUC	Comments
Doehner et al,[73] 2012	Prospective observational, single center	189	Acute stroke	Mortality, MACE, Rankin score	Mortality: HR 4.52 (1.1–19) MACE: HR 6.65 (1.8–24.9)	PENK not associated with renal function
Ng et al,[71] 2014	Prospective cohort, single center	1141	Unselected acute MI	Composite of death, reinfarction, heart failure hospitalization	All events: HR 1.52 (1.19–1.94) Death/MI: HR 1.76 (1.34–2.3) Death/HF: HR 1.67 (1.24–2.25) Recurrent MI: HR 1.43 (1.07–1.91)	PENK related to eGFR, LVWMI, sex, BP, age
Shah et al,[69] 2015	Post-hoc analysis, single center	92	Undergoing cardiac surgery	Acute kidney injury	OR 23.8 (2–270)	PENK strong correlation with creatinine
Marino et al,[70] 2015	Observational retrospective, single center	101	Consecutive attendances for suspected sepsis in ED	AKI and mortality at 7 d	AUC for AKI = 0.815 AUC for 7-d mortality = 0.69	PENK inversely correlated with creatinine clearance
Van Hateren et al,[76] 2015	Prospective observational, ZODIAC study	1157	Diabetic population	Cardiovascular mortality	HR 0.49 (1–1.21); no added predictive value	PENK correlates with creatinine
Melander et al,[75] 2015	(1) Malmo Diet and Cancer Study and (2) Malmo Preventive Project	(1) 1929 (2) 1569	Healthy population	Incidence of breast cancer	(1) HR 0.72 (0.62–0.85) (2) OR 0.63 (0.52–0.76)	PENK not compared with renal function. Lower PENK associated with increased breast cancer incidence
Schulz et al,[72] 2017	Prospective cohort, Swedish population study	2568	Healthy population	Chronic kidney disease	OR 1.51 (1.18–1.94)	PENK correlates with creatinine

Abbreviations: AKI, acute kidney injury; AUC, area under the curve; BP, blood pressure; ED, emergency department; eGFR, estimated glomerular filtration rate; HF, heart failure; HR, hazard ratio; LVWMI, left ventricular wall motion index; MACE, major adverse cardiac events; MI, myocardial infarction; OR, odds ratio; PENK, proenkephalin; ZODIAC, zwolle outpatient diabetes project integrating available care.

Table 2
Summary of studies using PENK for prognosis in heart failure

Author	Type of Study	Number of Patients	Inclusion Criteria	End Point	HR (95% CI)	Comments
Arbit et al,[77] 2016	Prospective cohort, single center	200	ACC/AHA stages A and B	Cardiovascular-related hospital admission/death	3.0 (1.4–6.7)	PENK correlates with serum creatinine, eGFR, LVEF, hypertension, and diabetes
Matsue et al,[78] 2017	Retrospective study	1589	Acute heart failure	Death/heart failure rehospitalization/cardiovascular or renal rehospitalization	NA	PENK correlates with diabetes, creatinine, and BNP, RBF, and GFR
Ng et al,[79] 2017	Observational multicenter cohort study	1908	Acute heart failure	1-y all-cause mortality/in-hospital mortality/heart failure rehospitalization/in-hospital worsening renal function	1.27 (1.10–1.45)	PENK correlates with hypertension, IHD, HF, and renal impairment

Abbreviations: BNP, brain natriuretic peptide; GFR, glomerular filtration rate; IHD, ischemic heart disease; NA, not available; RBF, renal blood flow.

PROTECT (Placebo-Controlled Randomized Study of the Selective A1 Adenosine Receptor Antagonist Rolofylline for Patients Hospitalized With Acute Decompensated Heart Failure and Volume Overload to Assess Treatment Effect on Congestion and Renal Function) prognostic model were made, which included age, history of heart failure hospitalization, severity of peripheral edema, systolic blood pressure, serum sodium, blood urea nitrogen, creatinine, and albumin. Moreover, PENK level was positively correlated with albuminuria in the chronic heart failure cohort.[78] These findings reinforce that PENK may be a novel renal marker.

More recently, Ng and colleagues[79] measured PENK levels in patients with acute heart failure, in a multicenter, registrylike cohort study involving 1908 unselected patients presenting with acute heart failure in 3 European sites. The primary end point was 1-year all-cause mortality and secondary end points included in-hospital mortality, all-cause mortality or heart failure rehospitalization within 1 year, and in-hospital worsening renal function. Plasma PENK level was strongly correlated with renal function (eGFR). The findings in this study suggest that PENK levels have additive value in providing modest accuracy to predict worsening renal function, when added to a model that includes a history of renal impairment, systolic blood pressure, and plasma sodium level. PENK level was independently prognostic for worsening renal function and levels increased over time, whereas renal function deteriorated. During follow-up, PENK level was a strong independent predictor of mortality and death and/or heart failure for both short-term (3-month) and longer-term (1-year) follow-up. In addition, PENK levels independently predicted outcomes at 3 or 6 months and were independent predictors of in-hospital mortality, predominantly downclassifying risk in survivors when added to clinical scores; levels less than 133.3 pmol/L and greater than 211.3 pmol/L detected low-risk and high-risk patients, respectively. These PENK levels can be of use in making clinical decisions and predicting cardiorenal syndrome, which may allow selection of patients with acute heart failure for intensified therapy settings or ruling out such care in low-risk patients. In addition, improved risk prediction could facilitate decision making on the frequency of monitoring of renal function and rate of uptitration of heart failure therapies.[79] **Table 2** summarizes the studies that have used PENK for prognosis in heart failure. **Fig. 1** summarizes the role of proenkephalin in prognosis for patients with cardiovascular diseases.

DISCUSSION

The strong association between PENK level and renal function requires exploration, especially in light of the independent predictive value of PENK for mortality in heart failure, in addition to traditional risk markers and even after adjusting for renal function. Opioid agonist administration causes profound changes in renal excretory function.[80] δ-Opioid agonism increases both urinary water and sodium excretion, but lower doses of δ-opioid agonism only increase renal excretion of water. The use of the nonpeptide δ-opioid receptor agonist BW373U86 increases urine output without change to heart rate or blood pressure, an effect that is abolished by selective δ-opioid receptor antagonism. Like in the heart, these effects seem paired to sympathetic activation and innervation, because the diuretic effect was abolished in rats having undergone bilateral renal denervation,[81] although it is not clear at present whether this is caused by the loss of afferent or efferent innervation. Although other mechanisms contribute to water and salt homeostasis in heart failure, this link strengthens the likelihood of a direct proenkephalin-renal relationship.

SUMMARY

The enkephalin system plays a significant role in cardiovascular diseases. Plasma PENK, a stable and likely surrogate for mature intracellular enkephalin synthesis, has given new insight into mechanisms involved in various related cardiovascular diseases as well as the importance of the cardiorenal axis in prognosis in heart failure. PENK level could be just a surrogate for glomerular filtration rate. Being a stable and small peptide fragment (~ 4.5 kDa), it is likely that PENK is filtered by the kidneys, and PENK level has been shown to be associated with glomerular function, and not tubular function. However, because of the high density of δ-opioid receptors in the kidney, as well as the likely autocrine/paracrine nature of enkephalin signaling, enkephalins are likely to have a direct effect on kidneys, especially in heart failure. Sympathetic pathways could link the heart and kidneys in a feedback axis that involves the brain and adrenals, with the ultimate aim of increasing urine output, and increasing cardiac output in heart failure. The effect of opioid receptor stimulation in the heart on blood pressure and heart rate may be partially beneficial for reducing preload and afterload, but the reduction in myocardial contractility seems counterproductive, but may be cardioprotective overall. Whether any of these pathways can be exploited to improve outcome in heart failure requires further investigative work.

REFERENCES

1. van den Brink OW, Delbridge LM, Rosenfeldt FL, et al. Endogenous cardiac opioids: enkephalins in adaptation and protection of the heart. Heart Lung Circ 2003;12(3):178–87.

2. Kosterlitz HW, Hughes J. Some thoughts on the significance of enkephalin, the endogenous ligand. Life Sci 1975;17(1):91–6.

3. Hughes J, Smith TW, Kosterlitz HW, et al. Identification of two related pentapeptides from the brain with potent opiate agonist activity. Nature 1975; 258(5536):577–80.

4. Holaday JW. Cardiovascular effects of endogenous opiate systems. Annu Rev Pharmacol Toxicol 1983; 23:541–94.

5. Tang J, Yang HY, Costa E. Distribution of met5-enkephalin-Arg6-Phe7 (MEAP) in various tissues of rats and guinea pigs. Life Sci 1982;31(20–21): 2303–6.

6. Barron BA. Opioid peptides and the heart. Cardiovasc Res 1999;43(1):13–6.

7. Udenfriend S, Kilpatrick DL. Biochemistry of the enkephalins and enkephalin-containing peptides. Arch Biochem Biophys 1983;221(2):309–23.

8. Baker AK, Meert TF. Functional effects of systemically administered agonists and antagonists of mu, delta, and kappa opioid receptor subtypes on body temperature in mice. J Pharmacol Exp Ther 2002;302(3):1253–64.

9. Dhawan BN, Cesselin F, Raghubir R, et al. International union of pharmacology. XII. Classification of opioid receptors. Pharmacol Rev 1996;48(4):567–92.

10. Jackson KE, Farias M, Stanfill A, et al. Delta opioid receptors inhibit vagal bradycardia in the sinoatrial node. J Cardiovasc Pharmacol Ther 2001;6(4):385–93.

11. Stefano GB, Scharrer B, Smith EM, et al. Opioid and opiate immunoregulatory processes. Crit Rev Immunol 1996;16(2):109–44.

12. Tsao LI, Su TP. Hibernation-induction peptide and cell death: [D-Ala2,D-Leu5]enkephalin blocks Bax-related apoptotic processes. Eur J Pharmacol 2001;428(1):149–51.

13. Feuerstein G, Siren AL. The opioid system in cardiac and vascular regulation of normal and hypertensive states. Circulation 1987;75(1 Pt 2):I125–9.

14. Giles TD, Sander GE. Mechanism of the cardiovascular response to systemic intravenous administration of leucine-enkephalin in the conscious dog. Peptides 1983;4(2):171–5.

15. Ventura C, Capogrossi M, Lakatta E. Myocardial function and endogenous opioids. Clinical perspectives in endogenous opioid peptides. West Sussex, UK: John Wiley; 1992. p. 393–406.

16. Springhorn JP, Claycomb WC. Translation of heart preproenkephalin mRNA and secretion of enkephalin peptides from cultured cardiac myocytes. Am J Physiol 1992;263(5 Pt 2):H1560–6.

17. Wilson SP, Klein RL, Chang KJ, et al. Are opioid peptides co-transmitters in noradrenergic vesicles of sympathetic nerves? Nature 1980;288(5792):707–9.

18. Comb M, Seeburg PH, Adelman J, et al. Primary structure of the human Met- and Leu-enkephalin precursor and its mRNA. Nature 1982;295(5851):663–6.

19. Noda M, Furutani Y, Takahashi H, et al. Cloning and sequence analysis of cDNA for bovine adrenal preproenkephalin. Nature 1982;295(5846):202–6.

20. Beinfeld MC. Prohormone and proneuropeptide processing. Recent progress and future challenges. Endocrine 1998;8(1):1–5.

21. Howells RD, Kilpatrick DL, Bailey LC, et al. Proenkephalin mRNA in rat heart. Proc Natl Acad Sci U S A 1986;83(6):1960–3.

22. Low KG, Allen RG, Melner MH. Association of proenkephalin transcripts with polyribosomes in the heart. Mol Endocrinol 1990;4(9):1408–15.

23. Younes A, Pepe S, Barron BA, et al. Cardiac synthesis, processing, and coronary release of enkephalin-related peptides. Am J Physiol Heart Circ Physiol 2000;279(4):H1989–98.

24. Barron BA. Cardiac opioids. Proc Soc Exp Biol Med 2000;224(1):1–7.

25. Liston D, Patey G, Rossier J, et al. Processing of proenkephalin is tissue-specific. Science 1984; 225(4663):734–7.

26. Kerr MA, Kenny AJ. The purification and specificity of a neutral endopeptidase from rabbit kidney brush border. Biochem J 1974;137(3):477–88.

27. Malfroy B, Swerts JP, Guyon A, et al. High-affinity enkephalin-degrading peptidase in brain is increased after morphine. Nature 1978;276(5687):523–6.

28. Mosnaim AD, Puente J, Wolf ME, et al. Studies of the in vitro human plasma degradation of methionine-enkephalin. Gen Pharmacol 1988;19(5):729–33.

29. Piedimonte G, Nadel JA, Long CS, et al. Neutral endopeptidase in the heart. Neutral endopeptidase inhibition prevents isoproterenol-induced myocardial hypoperfusion in rats by reducing bradykinin degradation. Circ Res 1994;75(4):770–9.

30. De la Baume S, Brion F, Dam Trung Tuong M, et al. Evaluation of enkephalinase inhibition in the living mouse, using [3H]acetorphan as a probe. J Pharmacol Exp Ther 1988;247(2):653–60.

31. Murry CE, Jennings RB, Reimer KA. Preconditioning with ischemia: a delay of lethal cell injury in ischemic myocardium. Circulation 1986;74(5):1124–36.

32. Maslov LN, Lishmanov YB, Oeltgen PR, et al. Comparative analysis of the cardioprotective properties of opioid receptor agonists in a rat model of myocardial infarction. Acad Emerg Med 2010; 17(11):1239–46.

33. Schultz JE, Hsu AK, Gross GJ. Ischemic preconditioning in the intact rat heart is mediated by delta1- but not

mu- or kappa-opioid receptors. Circulation 1998; 97(13):1282–9.

34. Borges JP, Verdoorn KS, Daliry A, et al. Delta opioid receptors: the link between exercise and cardioprotection. PLoS One 2014;9(11):e113541.

35. Sato T, Marban E. The role of mitochondrial K(ATP) channels in cardioprotection. Basic Res Cardiol 2000;95(4):285–9.

36. Holmuhamedov EL, Wang L, Terzic A. ATP-sensitive K+ channel openers prevent Ca2+ overload in rat cardiac mitochondria. J Physiol 1999;519 Pt 2:347–60.

37. Cao Z, Liu L, Van Winkle DM. Activation of delta- and kappa-opioid receptors by opioid peptides protects cardiomyocytes via KATP channels. Am J Physiol Heart Circ Physiol 2003;285(3):H1032–9.

38. Karck M, Tanaka S, Bolling SF, et al. Myocardial protection by ischemic preconditioning and delta-opioid receptor activation in the isolated working rat heart. J Thorac Cardiovasc Surg 2001;122(5): 986–92.

39. Tomai F, Crea F, Gaspardone A, et al. Effects of naloxone on myocardial ischemic preconditioning in humans. J Am Coll Cardiol 1999;33(7):1863–9.

40. Kevelaitis E, Peynet J, Mouas C, et al. Opening of potassium channels: the common cardioprotective link between preconditioning and natural hibernation? Circulation 1999;99(23):3079–85.

41. Prasad SK, Clerk A, Cullingford TE, et al. Gene expression profiling of human hibernating myocardium: increased expression of B-type natriuretic peptide and proenkephalin in hypocontractile vs normally-contracting regions of the heart. Eur J Heart Fail 2008;10(12):1177–80.

42. Zagon IS, Ruth TB, Leure-duPree AE, et al. Immunoelectron microscopic localization of the opioid growth factor receptor (OGFr) and OGF in the cornea. Brain Res 2003;967(1–2):37–47.

43. Zagon IS, Sassani JW, Allison G, et al. Conserved expression of the opioid growth factor, [Met5] enkephalin, and the zeta (zeta) opioid receptor in vertebrate cornea. Brain Res 1995;671(1):105–11.

44. Zagon IS, Verderame MF, Zimmer WE, et al. Molecular characterization and distribution of the opioid growth factor receptor (OGFr) in mouse. Brain Res Mol Brain Res 2000;84(1–2):106–14.

45. Zagon IS, Gibo DM, McLaughlin PJ. Ontogeny of zeta (zeta), the opioid growth factor receptor, in the rat brain. Brain Res 1992;596(1–2):149–56.

46. Zagon IS, Verderame MF, Allen SS, et al. Cloning, sequencing, chromosomal location, and function of cDNAs encoding an opioid growth factor receptor (OGFr) in humans. Brain Res 2000;856(1–2):75–83.

47. Uhlen M, Fagerberg L, Hallstrom BM, et al. Proteomics. Tissue-based map of the human proteome. Science 2015;347(6220):1260419.

48. McTavish N, Copeland LA, Saville MK, et al. Proenkephalin assists stress-activated apoptosis through transcriptional repression of NF-kappaB- and p53-regulated gene targets. Cell Death Differ 2007; 14(9):1700–10.

49. Liang CS, Imai N, Stone CK, et al. The role of endogenous opioids in congestive heart failure: effects of nalmefene on systemic and regional hemodynamics in dogs. Circulation 1987;75(2):443–51.

50. Imai N, Kashiki M, Woolf PD, et al. Comparison of cardiovascular effects of mu- and delta-opioid receptor antagonists in dogs with congestive heart failure. Am J Physiol 1994;267(3 Pt 2):H912–7.

51. Kho C, Lee A, Hajjar RJ. Altered sarcoplasmic reticulum calcium cycling–targets for heart failure therapy. Nat Rev Cardiol 2012;9(12):717–33.

52. Ding YF, Brower GL, Zhong Q, et al. Defective intracellular Ca2+ homeostasis contributes to myocyte dysfunction during ventricular remodelling induced by chronic volume overload in rats. Clin Exp Pharmacol Physiol 2008;35(7):827–35.

53. Xiao RP, Pepe S, Spurgeon HA, et al. Opioid peptide receptor stimulation reverses beta-adrenergic effects in rat heart cells. Am J Physiol 1997;272(2 Pt 2): H797–805.

54. Ela C, Barg J, Vogel Z, et al. Distinct components of morphine effects on cardiac myocytes are mediated by the kappa and delta opioid receptors. J Mol Cell Cardiol 1997;29(2):711–20.

55. Treskatsch S, Feldheiser A, Shaqura M, et al. Cellular localization and adaptive changes of the cardiac delta opioid receptor system in an experimental model of heart failure in rats. Heart Vessels 2016;31(2):241–50.

56. Pepe S, Xiao RP, Hohl C, et al. 'Cross talk' between opioid peptide and adrenergic receptor signaling in isolated rat heart. Circulation 1997;95(8):2122–9.

57. Sakamoto S, Liang CS. Opiate receptor inhibition improves the blunted baroreflex function in conscious dogs with right-sided congestive heart failure. Circulation 1989;80(4):1010–5.

58. Kawashima S, Fukutake N, Nishian K, et al. Elevated plasma beta-endorphin levels in patients with congestive heart failure. J Am Coll Cardiol 1991; 17(1):53–8.

59. Fontana F, Bernardi P, Pich EM, et al. Relationship between plasma atrial natriuretic factor and opioid peptide levels in healthy subjects and in patients with acute congestive heart failure. Eur Heart J 1993;14(2):219–25.

60. Peacock WF, Hollander JE, Diercks DB, et al. Morphine and outcomes in acute decompensated heart failure: an ADHERE analysis. Emerg Med J 2008;25(4):205–9.

61. Fricker LD, Supattapone S, Snyder SH. Enkephalin convertase: a specific enkephalin synthesizing carboxypeptidase in adrenal chromaffin granules, brain, and pituitary gland. Life Sci 1982;31(16–17): 1841–4.

62. Birch NP, Christie DL. Characterization of the molecular forms of proenkephalin in bovine adrenal medulla and rat adrenal, brain, and spinal cord with a site-directed antiserum. J Biol Chem 1986;261(26):12213–21.

63. Fleminger G, Ezra E, Kilpatrick DL, et al. Processing of enkephalin-containing peptides in isolated bovine adrenal chromaffin granules. Proc Natl Acad Sci U S A 1983;80(20):6418–21.

64. Wilson SP. Purification of peptides derived from proenkephalin A on Bio-Rex 70. J Neurosci Methods 1985;15(2):155–63.

65. Ernst A, Kohrle J, Bergmann A. Proenkephalin A 119-159, a stable proenkephalin A precursor fragment identified in human circulation. Peptides 2006;27(7):1835–40.

66. Datar P, Srivastava S, Coutinho E, et al. structure, function, and therapeutics. Curr Top Med Chem 2004;4(1):75–103.

67. Harrison S, Geppetti P. Substance p. Int J Biochem Cell Biol 2001;33(6):555–76.

68. Ernst A, Buerger K, Hartmann O, et al. Midregional proenkephalin A and N-terminal protachykinin A are decreased in the cerebrospinal fluid of patients with dementia disorders and acute neuroinflammation. J Neuroimmunol 2010;221(1–2):62–7.

69. Shah KS, Taub P, Patel M, et al. Proenkephalin predicts acute kidney injury in cardiac surgery patients. Clin Nephrol 2015;83(1):29–35.

70. Marino R, Struck J, Hartmann O, et al. Diagnostic and short-term prognostic utility of plasma proenkephalin (pro-ENK) for acute kidney injury in patients admitted with sepsis in the emergency department. J Nephrol 2015;28(6):717–24.

71. Ng LL, Sandhu JK, Narayan H, et al. Proenkephalin and prognosis after acute myocardial infarction. J Am Coll Cardiol 2014;63(3):280–9.

72. Schulz CA, Christensson A, Ericson U, et al. High level of fasting plasma proenkephalin-A predicts deterioration of kidney function and incidence of CKD. J Am Soc Nephrol 2017;28(1):291–303.

73. Doehner W, von Haehling S, Suhr J, et al. Elevated plasma levels of neuropeptide proenkephalin a predict mortality and functional outcome in ischemic stroke. J Am Coll Cardiol 2012;60(4):346–54.

74. Denning GM, Ackermann LW, Barna TJ, et al. Proenkephalin expression and enkephalin release are widely observed in non-neuronal tissues. Peptides 2008;29(1):83–92.

75. Melander O, Orho-Melander M, Manjer J, et al. Stable peptide of the endogenous opioid enkephalin precursor and breast cancer risk. J Clin Oncol 2015;33(24):2632–8.

76. van Hateren KJ, Landman GW, Arnold JF, et al. Serum proenkephalin A levels and mortality after long-term follow-up in patients with type 2 diabetes mellitus (ZODIAC-32). PLoS One 2015;10(7):e0133065.

77. Arbit B, Marston N, Shah K, et al. Prognostic usefulness of proenkephalin in stable ambulatory patients with heart failure. Am J Cardiol 2016;117(8):1310–4.

78. Matsue Y, Ter Maaten JM, Struck J, et al. Clinical correlates and prognostic value of proenkephalin in acute and chronic heart failure. J Card Fail 2017;23(3):231–9.

79. Ng LL, Squire IB, Jones DJ, et al. Proenkephalin, renal dysfunction, and prognosis in patients with acute heart failure: a GREAT Network Study. J Am Coll Cardiol 2017;69(1):56–69.

80. Kapusta DR. Opioid mechanisms controlling renal function. Clin Exp Pharmacol Physiol 1995;22(12):891–902.

81. Sezen SF, Kenigs VA, Kapusta DR. Renal excretory responses produced by the delta opioid agonist, BW373U86, in conscious rats. J Pharmacol Exp Ther 1998;287(1):238–45.

Natriuretic Peptides in Heart Failure
Atrial and B-type Natriuretic Peptides

Alan S. Maisel, MD[a],*, Jason M. Duran, MD, PhD[b],
Nicholas Wettersten, MD[c]

KEYWORDS

- B-type natriuretic peptide • N-terminal B-type natriuretic peptide
- Midregional pro–atrial natriuretic peptide • Heart failure • Diagnosis • Prognosis

KEY POINTS

- The natriuretic peptides are important biomarkers for diagnosing and risk stratifying patients with heart failure.
- B-type natriuretic peptide (BNP) and N-terminal proBNP (NT-proBNP) can help optimize therapy in patients with chronic heart failure.
- The natriuretic peptides also have an important use for prognostication in other cardiovascular diseases.
- Further research is needed to understand how to interpret BNP and NT-proBNP in the setting of new neprilysin inhibitors.

INTRODUCTION

The natriuretic peptides (NPs) play a critical role in maintaining homeostasis in the cardiovascular system, serving as counter-regulatory hormones for volume and pressure overload. It was recognized early that measurement of NPs might serve as useful surrogates for patient status and pathophysiology. With more than 3 decades of research, NPs are now vital tools in the diagnosis of heart failure (HF), can also aid in prognosis, and can sometimes help with guiding therapy. Their utility also extends beyond HF into other cardiovascular and noncardiovascular conditions. However, with the introduction of neprilysin inhibitors that alter the physiology of the NP system, a new avenue of research has opened to better understand the

changes that occur in clinical assessment of NPs. This article discusses the history and uses of NP assessment in HF and other cardiovascular diseases.

Physiologic Production of the Natriuretic Peptides

The existence of atrial NP (ANP), also known as atrial natriuretic factor, was first recognized in 1981 when homogenized atrial tissues were injected into rats and resulted in a reduction of blood pressure, diuresis, and natriuresis.[1] Subsequent research led to a further understanding of the NP system and the discovery of B-type natriuretic peptide (BNP), also known as brain-type natriuretic peptide, and C-type natriuretic peptide

Disclosures: Dr A.S. Maisel has ongoing research projects with Abbott and Roche, and he does consulting for Alere. J.M. Duran and N. Wettersten have no disclosures.
[a] Division of Cardiovascular Medicine, VA San Diego Healthcare System 111-A, 3350 La Jolla Village Drive, San Diego, CA 92161, USA; [b] Department of Internal Medicine, UC San Diego, 200 West Arbor Drive, La Jolla, San Diego, CA 92103, USA; [c] Division of Cardiovascular Medicine, UC San Diego, 9500 Gilman Drive MC 7411, La Jolla, San Diego, CA 92037-7411, USA
* Corresponding author.
E-mail address: amaisel@ucsd.edu

(CNP). At present, clinical assays for ANP and BNP are most widely used in cardiovascular disease and are discussed here.

ANP is encoded by the *NPAA* gene on chromosome 1. It is translated into a 151-amino-acid pre-prohormone (preproANP) that is cleaved in the sarcoplasmic reticulum to a 126-amino-acid pro-hormone (proANP), which is stored in intracellular granules.[2] When stimulated and released, proANP is further cleaved into a 28-amino-acid bioactive form (ANP) and a 98-amino-acid N-terminal fragment (NT-proANP).[2] The half-life of ANP is approximately 2 minutes, whereas NT-proANP half-life is variable depending on the fragment measured.[2]

ANP is predominantly produced in the atria of the heart and to a lesser extent the ventricles and extracardiac tissues, such as the kidney.[3] Unlike BNP, which has minimal preformed and stored hormone, most proANP is stored in intracellular granules of the atria and released on stimulation, whereas further production of ANP involves the slower process of transcription and translation.[4] The major stimulus for ANP release is increased atrial wall stretch reflecting increased intravascular volume. Other stimuli for release include catecholamines, arginine vasopressin, and endothelin.[3] These stimuli reflect the counter-regulatory role ANP plays against volume overload and hypertension.

BNP was first described in 1988 after isolation from porcine brain tissues (hence its original name of brain-type natriuretic peptide) with subsequent studies finding it produced in the cardiac ventricles.[5] As with ANP, BNP is a peptide neuro-hormone synthesized by cardiac ventricular myocytes in response to mechanical stretch.[6,7] During periods of volume overload, mechanical stretch on cardiomyocyte membranes activates signal transduction leading to downstream transcription and translation of preproBNP, a 134 amino acid precursor peptide.[8] PreproBNP undergoes a 2-step enzymatic cleavage to produce the biologically active product. The first cleavage occurs in the sarcoplasmic reticulum during translation, removing a 26-amino-acid signaling peptide and producing $proBNP_{1-108}$.[9,10] ProBNP subsequently undergoes a second cleavage by prohormone convertases (including the enzymes corin and furin) to produce the biologically active C-terminal peptide, BNP_{1-32}, and an inactive N-terminal fragment, NT-proBNP.[9] BNP and NT-proBNP peptides are secreted in equal concentrations into the circulation.[11-13] As discussed earlier, ANP is predominantly stored preformed in intracellular granules, but BNP is minimally stored and is mostly produced and secreted directly in large bursts following stimulation.[14] BNP has a

serum half-life of 20 minutes, whereas NT-proBNP has a half-life of 120 minutes (**Fig. 1**).[11,15]

ANP and BNP interact with 3 NP receptors (NPRs; A, B, and C) with their main physiologic effects exerted through the NPR-A receptor. The NPR-A receptor is the predominant form on blood vessels, with a smaller amount of NPR-B receptor, and both receptors are found in the kidneys and adrenal glands.[3] ANP and BNP binding to NPR-A and NPR-B leads to activation of guanylyl cyclase and downstream signaling through cyclic guanosine monophosphate (cGMP).[3] NPR-C clears ANP, and, to a lesser extent, BNP by binding and internalizing the receptor, and degrading the hormone. ANP is also inactivated and cleared by neutral endopeptidases (see **Fig. 1**).[2]

ANP signaling leads to a reduction in blood pressure, natriuresis, and diuresis. These actions are predominantly performed via effects on the kidneys. ANP increases renal blood flow, dilates afferent arterioles, and constricts efferent arterioles, leading to increased glomerular filtration.[16] It inhibits angiotensin II–mediated sodium and water reabsorption in the proximal tubule, inhibits sodium reabsorption in the inner medullary ducts, and antagonizes vasopressin, leading to decreased water reabsorption in the collecting duct.[17-20] These effects lead to a potent diuresis and natriuresis. Outside of the kidney, ANP reduces blood pressure by decreasing sympathetic output, increasing venous capacitance, and increasing vascular permeability.[21-23] These actions seem to be mediated by ANP inhibiting catecholamines, renin, angiotensin II, aldosterone, and endothelin.[24-28] ANP also directly affects the heart, preventing hypertrophy.[2]

When BNP circulates and binds NPRs on target tissues, it triggers increased intracellular cGMP signaling cascades, inducing actions that reduce cardiac preload and afterload to counteract the detrimental effects of pressure and volume overload, as seen in HF (see **Fig. 1**).[29] This process includes vasodilation, diuresis, natriuresis, and inhibition of the renin-angiotensin-aldosterone system (RAAS).[11] BNP is primarily cleared through degradation by circulating neutral endopeptidases and, to a lesser extent, through uptake by NPR-C in peripheral tissues and minimally through renal excretion (see **Fig. 1**).[11,29] These physiologic processes are counter-regulatory to the detrimental neurohormonal activation of the sympathetic nervous system and RAAS in HF and are why ANP and BNP levels reflect HF severity.

Clinical Assessment of the Natriuretic Peptides

BNP and NT-proBNP are measured using standard immunoassays that are now widely available;

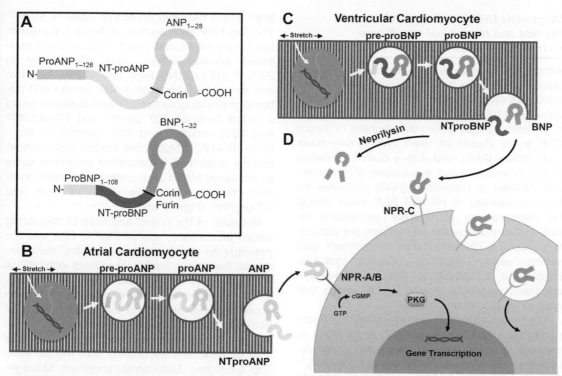

Fig. 1. ANP and BNP physiology. (*A*) Molecular structure of ANP (*top*) and BNP (*bottom*) showing enzymatic cleavage sites and end-product fragments. (*B*) Production and processing of ANP by atrial cardiac myocyte in response to mechanical stretch stimulus. (*C*) Production and processing of BNP by ventricular cardiac myocyte in response to mechanical stimulus. (*D*) Effects of ANP and BNP on target tissues. Both ANP and BNP bind NP receptor (NPR)A and NPR-B on target cells, inducing cleavage of guanosine triphosphate (GTP) to cyclic guanosine monophosphate (cGMP) by cytoplasmic G proteins, initiating an intracellular cGMP signaling cascade involving protein kinase G (PKG), ultimately leading to downstream transcription of genes involving smooth muscle cell relaxation, diuresis and natriuresis (depending on target tissue). Both ANP and BNP are broken down in serum by circulating endogenous peptidases, including neprilysin. ANP and BNP are also degraded (to a lesser extent) by cellular uptake through binding NPR-C, undergoing receptor-mediated endocytosis and intracellular breakdown by lysosomes.

however, they are controversial. The assays for detection of BNP rely on antibodies that have minimal cross-reactivity with NT-proBNP and vice versa.[30] The available BNP immunoassay relies on 2 monoclonal antibodies, recognizing the BNP ring structure and the C-terminal tail,[31] and these antibodies have significant cross-reactivity with portions of pro-BNP$_{1-108}$. Thus the available immunoassays measure total circulating BNP, including the biologically active BNP$_{1-32}$ and the inactive pro-BNP$_{1-108}$. The exact clinical significance of measuring the non–biologically active pro-BNP$_{1-108}$ remains unclear. Novel assays are now being developed that allow for differential measurement of BNP$_{1-32}$ and pro-BNP$_{1-108}$ isoforms.[32]

As mentioned, the bioactive form of ANP is labile with a very short half-life; thus, it is difficult to accurately measure the bioactive form in clinical practice.[33–35] As a result, the N-terminal

prohormone fragment (NT-proANP) was subsequently measured, which is more chemically stable in serum, but its concentrations may be higher than the bioactive isoform.[33] A variety of clinical assays, most often immunoassays, were developed to measure NT-proANP, but subsequently it was found that even the NT-proANP portion underwent further degradation.[33] In 2004, an assay was developed focusing on the midregion of NT-proANP (MR-proANP), because little proteolytic degradation occurs in this region.[33,36] MR-proANP is now the primary biomarker measured in clinical assays. Aside from MR-proANP, newer research has shown that fragments of the preprohormone may remain stable after cleavage and could be quantified, suggesting that assays could be developed to explore this marker of ANP physiology.[33] Further research is needed to establish whether this is a clinically useful marker.

Diagnostic Utility of B-type Natriuretic Peptide and N-terminal pro–B-type Natriuretic Peptide in Acute Heart Failure

Although the molecular structure and cellular production of BNP was first described in the late 1980s, its clinical significance was not fully elucidated until the early 2000s. The evidence is now overwhelming that early measurement of serum BNP levels should be used to diagnose acute heart failure (AHF), and it is a class I indication in the American Heart Association (AHA)/American College of Cardiology (ACC) guidelines for the management of HF that BNP levels should be measured in all hospital admissions for AHF.[37] Cardiac-specific biomarkers are particularly useful in the emergency department (ED) setting when evaluating dyspneic patients, because it is difficult to distinguish between shortness of breath caused by HF versus that caused by pulmonary disease.

The Breathing Not Properly Multinational Study published in 2002 was the first large study to evaluate the efficacy of BNP as a cardiac biomarker for diagnosis of HF in the ED setting.[14] This study evaluated 1586 patients presenting to EDs with the chief complaint of dyspnea at 7 different medical centers around the world. Serum BNP levels were higher in patients presenting with dyspnea caused by AHF than in dyspnea from a noncardiac cause. Serum BNP levels were positively correlated with severity of HF using the New York Heart Association (NYHA) classification. Using a BNP cutoff of 100 pg/mL, serum BNP level was 90% sensitive and 76% specific for HF. Using a cutoff of 50 pg/mL,

BNP had a negative predictive value of 96%.[14] The Pro-BNP Investigation of Acute Dyspnea in the Emergency Department (PRIDE) study published similar findings using NT-proBNP in 2005.[38] NT-proBNP level was highly sensitive and specific at diagnosing AHF among 600 patients presenting to the ED with dyspnea using a cutoff level of 300 pg/mL, and NT-proBNP was 90% sensitive and 85% specific for diagnosis of AHF.[38] Numerous studies have subsequently confirmed the excellent predictive value as assessed by the area under the receiver operator characteristic curve (AUC) of BNP and NT-proBNP (**Figs. 2** and **3**).

Because of the speed and ease of measuring serum biomarkers, use of BNP in EDs has the potential to greatly reduce hospital stay and overall treatment costs associated with HF. A 2004 study by Mueller and colleagues[39] evaluated 452 patients presenting to the ED with acute dyspnea and found that measurement of BNP led to more rapid HF diagnosis, which reduced time to discharge and decreased overall cost of treatment associated with the ED visit. The Canadian Multicenter Improved Management of Patients With Congestive Heart Failure (IMPROVE-CHF) study showed similar findings using NT-proBNP in a population of 500 patients presenting to 7 different EDs in Canada. Measurement of serum NT-proBNP level to aid in the diagnosis of HF reduced duration of ED visits by 21%, reduced the rate of rehospitalization after 60 days by 45%, and similarly reduced the overall cost of treatment of these patients.[40]

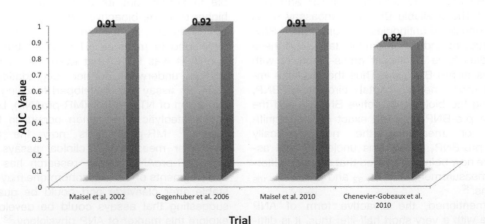

Fig. 2. Values for AUCs from major trials evaluating the predictive value of BNP, which show the excellent predictive value of BNP.

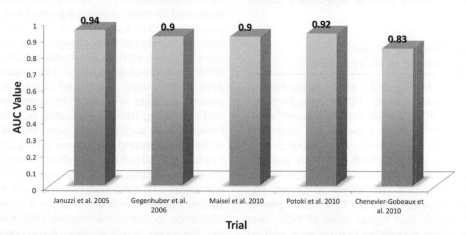

Fig. 3. Values for AUCs from major trials evaluating the predictive value of NT-proBNP, which show an excellent predictive value similar to BNP.

Diagnostic Utility Midregion Pro–Atrial Natriuretic Peptide in Acute Heart Failure

The largest study to evaluate MR-proANP for the diagnosis of AHF, the Biomarkers in Acute Heart Failure (BACH) study was a multisite international trial enrolling 1641 patients presenting with acute dyspnea, of whom 568 patients were diagnosed with AHF.[41] MR-proANP was noninferior to BNP and NT-proBNP with a sensitivity of 97.0%, a negative predictive value of 97.4% at a cutoff of 120 pmol/L, and an excellent AUC of 0.90.[41] Furthermore, the addition of MR-proANP to BNP improved the diagnostic performance of BNP

with the C-statistic increasing from 0.787 to 0.816, and it had an incremental benefit in diagnosing AHF in patients with BNP and NT-proBNP values in the gray zone as well as in obese patients.[41] Other studies have shown similar findings and furthered the evidence for MR-proANP for AHF (**Fig. 4**).[42–45] Similar improvements in the diagnosis of patients with AHF with BNP or NT-proBNP levels in the gray zone by MR-proANP have been found.[43] MR-proANP and BNP diagnosed AHF better than 8 other biomarkers.[42] The investigators of the PRIDE study explored different age-based cutoffs for MR-proANP (similar to NT-proBNP), which improved specificity

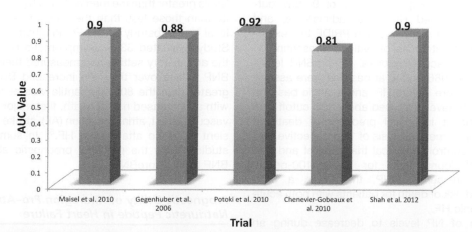

Fig. 4. Values for AUCs from major trials evaluating the predictive value of MR-proANP, again showing an excellent predictive value, as with BNP and NT-proBNP.

but decreased sensitivity.[44] Further study is needed to establish whether age-based cutoffs are indicated.

Prognostic Utility of B-type Natriuretic Peptide in Heart Failure

In addition to its diagnostic value, many studies have now shown the utility of BNP levels for prognostication. In 2002, Berger and colleagues[46] evaluated 452 ambulatory patients to determine whether serum BNP levels were predictive of future sudden cardiac death (SCD) in patients with a left ventricular ejection fraction (LVEF) less than 35% within a 3-year follow-up period. Patients with a baseline serum BNP level greater than 130 pg/mL had higher rates of SCD, and the investigators suggested that patients with an increased BNP level at baseline should be evaluated for implantable cardiac defibrillator therapy.[46] A substudy of the A Randomized Trial of the Angiotensin-Receptor Blocker Valsartan in Chronic Heart Failure (Val-HeFT) trial also evaluated the prognostic value of BNP.[47] This analysis was of 4300 patients who had serial serum BNP levels drawn at baseline, 4 months, and 12 months after enrollment. Patients with the largest percentage decline in BNP level from baseline during follow-up had the lowest morbidity and mortality. In contrast, patients with the highest percentage increase in BNP from baseline had the worst morbidity and mortality using a Cox proportional hazard model.[47]

The 2004 Rapid Emergency Department Heart Failure Outpatients Trial (REDHOT) trial evaluated 464 patients presenting to the ED with dyspnea and with NYHA class II to IV HF with baseline BNP greater than 100 pg/mL. The investigators found that baseline BNP levels greater than 200 pg/mL were strongly predictive of 90-day outcomes (combined HF visits, admissions, and mortality).[48] An analysis of the PRIDE trial examined 1-year outcomes of patients presenting to the ED with acute dyspnea. NT-proBNP levels greater than 986 pg/mL at baseline were associated with more severe HF, and a single baseline NT-proBNP level increased above this cutoff was the strongest individual predictor of death at 1 year.[49] In a meta-analysis of 19 prospective randomized controlled clinical trials, Doust and colleagues[50] found that, for every 100-pg/mL increase in serum BNP, there was a 35% increased risk of death for patients with both acute and chronic HF.

Failure of NP levels to decrease during an HF hospitalization while undergoing treatment is associated with worse prognosis and suggests a potential role for serial BNP measurement during HF hospitalization.[51,52] Cheng and colleagues[52] evaluated 72 male veterans admitted with decompensated NYHA class III to IV HF and followed them for 30 days after discharge. Serial BNP levels were followed, starting with baseline values drawn within 24 hours of admission. Of these patients, 13 died and 9 were readmitted during the study period. Patients who died or were readmitted had increasing BNP levels during hospitalization. Patients who survived and were not readmitted showed decreasing BNP levels during admission. In a study of 50 patients admitted for AHF, Bettencourt and colleagues[51] measured BNP levels at admission and then serially throughout hospitalization. Patients were followed for 6 months after discharge to determine whether BNP trends during the index hospitalization were predictive of end points including readmission for cardiovascular causes and death. Patients who died or were readmitted had less marked decline in BNP levels during hospitalization (770 ± 608 pg/mL to 643 ± 465 pg/mL; P = .08), whereas increasing BNP levels during hospitalization were associated with increased event rate (hazard ratio = 3.3; 95% confidence interval, 1.3–8.8).

Several large clinical databases have also been evaluated to determine the prognostic value of BNP in treatment of HF. In the Acute Decompensated Heart Failure National Registry (ADHERE) database of 65,275 patients with AHF, increased serum BNP levels at time of admission for HF exacerbation correlated with an increased risk of in-hospital mortality.[53] In a study of the Get With the Guidelines Heart Failure Registry, 99,930 patients with AHF were stratified into subgroups based on gender and LVEF (reduced, <40%; borderline, 40%–49%; preserved, ≥50%). Regardless of gender or LVEF, patients with BNP levels greater than the median had a higher mortality than those less than the median serum BNP level.[54] A substudy of the Framingham Offspring Study evaluated 3346 asymptomatic patients in the ambulatory setting and measured their serum BNP values over time. An increased BNP level greater than the 80th percentile was associated with an increased risk of death, first major cardiovascular event, atrial fibrillation (AF), stroke or transient ischemic attack, and HF.[55] In sum, these studies show the powerful prognostic ability of BNP and NT-proBNP.

Prognostic Utility of Midregion Pro–Atrial Natriuretic Peptide in Heart Failure

MR-proANP has shown significant prognostic utility for morbidity and mortality in acute and chronic

HF. Multiple studies have shown that increasing levels of MR-proANP are associated with increasing mortality in patients with AHF up to 4 years from presentation.[44,45,56] Findings are similar in chronic HF, with MR-proANP predictive of mortality more than 5 years after initial assessment.[45,57–59] Some studies have shown that serial monitoring of MR-proANP in chronic HF improves mortality prediction.[58,60] MR-proANP levels are also associated with risk of cardiovascular admission.[58]

MR-proANP has prognostic utility in non-HF cardiovascular conditions as well. In acute coronary syndrome, MR-proANP was highly predictive for mortality to the same degree as NT-proBNP, and combining both biomarkers captured more patients at risk for mortality.[61] In patients with stable coronary artery disease in the Prevention of Events With Angiotensin Converting Enzyme (PEACE) trial, MR-proANP levels were shown to risk stratify for the development of cardiovascular death and incident HF.[62] A biomarker substudy of the Rule Out Myocardial Infarction Using Computer Assisted Tomography (ROMICAT) trial showed that MR-proANP correlated with left atrial volume measured by cardiac computed tomography, suggesting MR-proANP can potentially screen for structural heart disease.[63] An analysis of the PRIDE study examining all patients presenting with dyspnea showed that MR-proANP had good prognostic utility for mortality up to 4 years from presentation.[44]

Some studies have also suggested that MR-proANP can serve as a screening tool in asymptomatic at-risk patients. In a large community-based population from Sweden, MR-proANP predicted incident HF and AF.[64] Although NT-proBNP and MR-proANP both predicted incident HF, only MR-proANP predicted incident AF.[64] In a study of men in Italy without known cardiovascular disease, NT-proANP (note: not MR-proANP assay) correlated better with risk prediction scores for cardiovascular outcomes than NT-proBNP because increasing tertiles of NT-proANP correlated with higher risk scores.[65] However, a limitation of this study was the use NT-proANP and not the more stable isoform MR-proANP, and levels were compared with risk scores rather than cardiovascular outcomes.

Using Serum Natriuretic Peptides to Guide Heart Failure Treatment

Whenever a patient is admitted for an HF exacerbation, the patient should have serum BNP level measured in the ED on admission, and this value should be compared with the baseline outpatient serum BNP level from when the patient was euvolemic, if available.[66] Several studies (as mentioned earlier) have suggested that BNP should then be trended during the course of hospitalization to help guide clinical management. In 2001, Kazanegra and colleagues[67] measured serial serum BNP levels and pulmonary capillary wedge pressures using Swan-Ganz catheters in patients admitted to the hospital for an AHF exacerbation. Treatment-related decreases in pulmonary capillary wedge pressures corresponded with declining serum BNP levels, suggesting that BNP levels should decline with diuresis. Although it may not be necessary to trend BNP levels daily in admitted patients, serial measurements should be considered in patients without clinical improvement to help guide therapy.

Several studies have shown that using a BNP-guided treatment strategy in outpatients with chronic HF translates into improved patient outcomes. The Plasma Brain Natriuretic Peptide-Guided Therapy to Improve Outcome in Heart Failure (STARS-BNP) trial published in 2007 evaluated the use of BNP-guided treatment strategies compared with standard clinical therapy in 220 patients with NYHA class II to III HF who were taking optimal medical management (angiotensin-converting enzyme [ACE] inhibitors, β-blockers, and diuretics).[68] Patients were randomized to receive BNP-guided treatment with a goal BNP level of less than 100 pg/mL or treatment guided by clinical and symptomatic improvement. By 15-month follow-up, patients in the BNP-guided treatment arm had a significantly lower primary outcome of HF-related death or readmission (24% vs 52%; $P<.001$).[68] The 2009 NT-proBNP–Assisted Treatment To Lessen Serial Cardiac Readmissions and Death (BATTLESCARRED) trial found similar results using NT-proBNP–guided clinical management.[69] In this trial, 364 patients admitted for HF exacerbation were assigned to NT-proBNP–guided therapy, intensive clinical management (using aggressive uptitration of HF medications to optimal clinical trial doses), or usual care using symptom-guided management. At 1-year follow-up, mortality was significantly lower in the NT-proBNP–guided treatment arm versus usual care (9.1% vs 18.9%; $P = .03$). By 3-year follow-up, mortality was significantly lower in the NT-proBNP–guided group (15.5%) compared with the intensive clinical management group (30.9%; $P = .048$) and usual-care group (31.3%; $P = .021$).[69] The 2009 Trial of Intensified versus Standard Medical Therapy in Elderly Patients With Congestive Heart Failure (TIME-CHF) study also evaluated NT-proBNP–guided therapy.[70] This trial included 499 patients with chronic HF who were older than 60 years, NYHA class greater than II, hospitalized for HF within the last year, and had a baseline NT-proBNP level greater than twice the upper limit of normal. These patients were followed for 18 months after initial admission, and the NT-proBNP–guided therapy arm had higher rates of survival and lower rates of all-cause hospitalizations in patients aged 60 to 75 years (P<.02) but not in patients older than 75 years (P<.02).[70] In addition, a 2014 meta-analysis by Troughton and colleagues[71] evaluated BNP-guided treatment in 2000 patients with HF and confirmed that BNP-guided treatment reduced all-cause mortality in patients less than 75 years old. Furthermore, BNP-guided treatment reduced hospitalizations caused by HF and cardiovascular disorders in all patients regardless of age or LVEF.[71]

MR-proANP has not been studied to the same extent as BNP or NT-proBNP for guiding therapy in HF or other conditions; however, some studies have suggested that it could be as useful. In a biomarker substudy of the PEACE trial, MR-proANP was one of 3 biomarkers showing an association between biomarkers levels and response to therapy with trandolapril.[62] If subjects had 2 or more of the biomarkers at increased levels, patients had an almost 50% reduction in cardiovascular death and incident HF with trandolapril, whereas subjects with none or 1 increased biomarker level did not derive benefit.[62] Another small study has suggested that MR-proANP can predict responsiveness to cardiac resynchronization therapy (CRT).[72] Patients who responded to CRT had lower MR-proANP levels at device insertion and levels decreased at 6 months compared with increased levels in nonresponders. Comparatively, midregional proadrenomedullin levels were lower at baseline in responders versus nonresponders, but levels did not change based on response at 6-month follow-up. NT-proBNP levels showed a trend to lower levels in responders versus nonresponders at baseline but decreased in both groups at 6-month follow-up. Increased levels of all 3 biomarkers were associated with higher rates of major adverse cardiovascular events at 2 years. Further studies are needed to establish whether MR-proANP can reproduce or enhance the findings that BNP and NT-proBNP have had at guiding treatment in HF.

Limitations of Natriuretic Peptide Measurement

There are several factors that can increase baseline serum NP levels, including age, female gender, and renal dysfunction. Higher baseline levels of BNP have been observed with increasing age; however, the exact mechanism is unknown.[73] This age-related increase was independent of age-related diastolic dysfunction. Some investigators have hypothesized that this is caused by reduced expression of NPRs with age, which could result in decreased clearance of circulating BNPs in older patients.[11] Several studies have shown that women have higher levels of BNP and NT-proBNP.[73,74] These studies evaluated age-matched cohorts in which serum BNP and NT-proBNP levels were higher in women than in men at any age, although the reason for this finding was not clear.[73,74] Some have proposed that estrogen levels may play a role in this observation, because women on hormone replacement therapy had higher baseline serum BNP levels than those not taking hormone therapy.[73] However, NT-proBNP levels were not increased in women on hormone replacement, making the role of estrogen in NP levels less clear. In addition, renal dysfunction may cause increases in baseline serum NP levels, but the reason for this is not clearly understood. BNP is primarily cleared from circulation through degradation by circulating endogenous peptidases rather than by renal clearance.[75] The mechanism behind this observation is probably multifactorial, considering that patients with renal dysfunction tend to be older and less healthy, with higher intravascular volume and ventricular strain contributing to increased baseline BNP levels independently of renal function.

In contrast, several factors may decrease baseline serum BNP levels, including obesity and flash pulmonary edema. Although obesity is a well-documented factor that can decrease baseline serum BNP level, the exact mechanism behind this remains unclear.[74,76–78] Adipocytes are known to have increased concentration of NPRs, thus obese patients may have greater clearance of BNP by adipocytes.[79] However, other studies have shown a correlation between BNP levels and lean mass rather than fat, which contradicts this hypothesis.[80] It is less clear whether serum NT-proBNP level is similarly decreased in obese patients, and, unlike BNP, NT-proBNP is not cleared by NPRs (natriuretic peptide receptors). Regardless, NT-proBNP retains its diagnostic value in obese patients as long as it is measured against a known baseline value.[80] In addition, patients with early flash pulmonary edema may have lower than expected serum BNP levels. As discussed earlier, volume overload produces mechanical stretch on cardiomyocyte cell membranes, leading to downstream transcription and translation of BNP. Flash pulmonary edema occurs so rapidly that BNP is not translated rapidly enough to be detected early in the disease course of these patients, making serum BNP less useful in this setting.[7]

Similar to BNP and NT-proBNP, certain caveats to MR-proANP interpretation should be noted. An analysis of the BACH study examined the influences of age, sex, race, and body mass index (BMI) on the diagnostic utility of MR-proANP and showed that it retained a high sensitivity regardless of these factors.[81] MR-proANP levels were noted to increase with age, decrease with BMI, and vary with race; however, a lower cutoff was only suggested for white patients younger than 50 years.[81] Other studies have confirmed the influence of BMI on MR-proANP levels.[58,82] In addition, levels go up with decreasing glomerular filtration rate (GFR), with one study suggesting potential adjustment in cutoffs based on GFR.[57,58,82,83] Overall, there are fewer studies evaluating factors influencing MR-proANP levels compared with studies for BNP and NT-proBNP, thus further study is needed to confirm these findings.

Measurement of B-type Natriuretic Peptide in Patients Taking Neprilysin Inhibitors

The 2014 Angiotensin–Neprilysin Inhibition versus Enalapril in Heart Failure (PARADIGM-HF) trial compared the novel neprilysin-angiotensin inhibitor LCZ696, a combination of the salt form of valsartan combined with sacubitril, with the ACE inhibitor enalapril and showed a dramatic improvement in the primary outcome of mortality and HF hospitalization with LCZ696.[84] Sacubitril is an inhibitor of neprilysin, a circulating neutral endopeptidase involved in the degradation of NPs.[85] As the clinical use of sacubitril-valsartan becomes more widespread, there is a growing concern that the measurement of serum NP levels in patients taking this drug may be problematic. In patients taking the neprilysin inhibitor, levels of BNP, which is broken down by neprilysin among other enzymes, may be increased because of decreased serum breakdown rather than because of change in underlying disease state (such as volume overload in AHF), potentially interfering with the prognostic and diagnostic utility of BNP.[86]

Results from the PARADIGM-HF trial did show that plasma BNP concentrations were significantly increased in patients taking sacubitril-valsartan versus enalapril, whereas NT-proBNP levels were significantly lower in the sacubitril-valsartan group.[87] However, the decreases were only modest and, although significantly different between the two treatment arms, the mean serum values in each group decreased to well within the anticipated variation of these biomarkers.[88,89] Neprilysin primarily breaks down ANP and CNP, whereas BNP may be more resistant to neprilysin cleavage.[90] As such, serum BNP levels may be less affected by neprilysin inhibition, as implied by initial interpretations of the PARADIGM-HF trial results.

Although more studies will be needed to determine the exact effect of neprilysin inhibition on BNP, there are some data to support that NT-proBNP may be more reliable in patients taking sacubitril.[86] The earlier Angiotensin Receptor Neprilysin Inhibitor LCZ696 in Heart Failure with Preserved Ejection Fraction (PARAMOUNT) trial examined effects of sacubitril-valsartan compared with valsartan alone in patients with chronic HF with preserved ejection fraction. Although significant early declines in NT-proBNP were observed at 12 weeks, NT-proBNP levels were no longer significantly different between the two groups after 36 weeks. Serum BNP was not measured in this trial.[91,92] At present, there are no published data on MR-proANP levels in patients taking sacubitril-valsartan.

SUMMARY

Since their discovery in the 1980s, extensive research has shown the important physiologic actions NPs play in regulating the detrimental neurohormonal effects occurring in patients with HF. Thus, they serve as an appropriate and excellent surrogate marker for assessing HF. A summary of the clinical applications of the NPs discussed is shown in **Table 1**. Ample evidence has shown

Table 1
Comparison of midregion of N-terminal Pro–atrial natriuretic peptide, B-type natriuretic peptide, and N-terminal pro–B-type natriuretic peptide in the management of heart failure

	MR-proANP	BNP	NT-proBNP
Diagnostic of HF?	+++	+++	+++
Prognostic of HF?	++	++	++
Levels Change with treatment	+/−	+++	++
Evidence for Guided Therapy	+/?	+/?	+/?
Levels affected by Entresto	?	+/?	—
Useful for outpatient screening?	+	+	+

the utility of BNP, NT-proBNP, and MR-proANP in the diagnosis of HF, leading to the ACC/AHA heart failure guidelines to give a class I recommendation to measurement of BNP or NT-proBNP in patients with AHF. Furthermore, there is considerable evidence showing the usefulness of NP for prognostication and guiding therapy. Also, the roles of NP assessment extend beyond HF to many other cardiovascular conditions. Although numerous clinical uses have been described for NPs, further roles are being explored in the prevention of HF and other cardiovascular and noncardiovascular conditions. Further research will surely expand the roles of NPs in the management of HF and other conditions.

REFERENCES

1. de Bold AJ, Borenstein HB, Veress AT, et al. A rapid and potent natriuretic response to intravenous injection of atrial myocardial extract in rats. Life Sci 1981; 28:89–94.
2. Volpe M, Carnovali M, Mastromarino V. The natriuretic peptides system in the pathophysiology of heart failure: from molecular basis to treatment. Clin Sci (Lond) 2016;130:57–77.
3. Levin ER, Gardner DG, Samson WK. Natriuretic peptides. N Engl J Med 1998;339:321–8.
4. Hall C. Essential biochemistry and physiology of (NT-pro)BNP. Eur J Heart Fail 2004;6:257–60.
5. Sudoh T, Minamino N, Kangawa K, et al. Brain natriuretic peptide-32: N-terminal six amino acid extended form of brain natriuretic peptide identified in porcine brain. Biochem Biophys Res Commun 1988;155:726–32.
6. Yasue H, Yoshimura M, Sumida H, et al. Localization and mechanism of secretion of B-type natriuretic peptide in comparison with those of A-type natriuretic peptide in normal subjects and patients with heart failure. Circulation 1994;90:195–203.
7. Yoshimura M, Yasue H, Okumura K, et al. Different secretion patterns of atrial natriuretic peptide and brain natriuretic peptide in patients with congestive heart failure. Circulation 1993;87:464–9.
8. Sudoh T, Maekawa K, Kojima M, et al. Cloning and sequence analysis of cDNA encoding a precursor for human brain natriuretic peptide. Biochem Biophys Res Commun 1989;159:1427–34.
9. Hammerer-Lercher A, Halfinger B, Sarg B, et al. Analysis of circulating forms of proBNP and NT-proBNP in patients with severe heart failure. Clin Chem 2008;54:858–65.
10. Semenov AG, Postnikov AB, Tamm NN, et al. Processing of pro-brain natriuretic peptide is suppressed by O-glycosylation in the region close to the cleavage site. Clin Chem 2009;55: 489–98.

11. Daniels LB, Maisel AS. Natriuretic peptides. J Am Coll Cardiol 2007;50:2357–68.
12. Nakagawa O, Ogawa Y, Itoh H, et al. Rapid transcriptional activation and early mRNA turnover of brain natriuretic peptide in cardiocyte hypertrophy. Evidence for brain natriuretic peptide as an "emergency" cardiac hormone against ventricular overload. J Clin Invest 1995;96:1280–7.
13. Kojima M, Minamino N, Kangawa K, et al. Cloning and sequence analysis of cDNA encoding a precursor for rat brain natriuretic peptide. Biochem Biophys Res Commun 1989;159:1420–6.
14. Maisel AS, Krishnaswamy P, Nowak RM, et al, Breathing Not Properly Multinational Study Investigators. Rapid measurement of B-type natriuretic peptide in the emergency diagnosis of heart failure. N Engl J Med 2002;347:161–7.
15. Maisel A, Mueller C, Adams K Jr, et al. State of the art: using natriuretic peptide levels in clinical practice. Eur J Heart Fail 2008;10:824–39.
16. Marin-Grez M, Fleming JT, Steinhausen M. Atrial natriuretic peptide causes pre-glomerular vasodilatation and post-glomerular vasoconstriction in rat kidney. Nature 1986;324:473–6.
17. Harris PJ, Thomas D, Morgan TO. Atrial natriuretic peptide inhibits angiotensin-stimulated proximal tubular sodium and water reabsorption. Nature 1987;326:697–8.
18. Dillingham MA, Anderson RJ. Inhibition of vasopressin action by atrial natriuretic factor. Science 1986;231:1572–3.
19. Zeidel ML. Regulation of collecting duct Na+ reabsorption by ANP 31-67. Clin Exp Pharmacol Physiol 1995;22:121–4.
20. Light DB, Corbin JD, Stanton BA. Dual ion-channel regulation by cyclic GMP and cyclic GMP-dependent protein kinase. Nature 1990;344:336–9.
21. Wijeyaratne CN, Moult PJ. The effect of alpha human atrial natriuretic peptide on plasma volume and vascular permeability in normotensive subjects. J Clin Endocrinol Metab 1993;76:343–6.
22. Schultz HD, Gardner DG, Deschepper CF, et al. Vagal C-fiber blockade abolishes sympathetic inhibition by atrial natriuretic factor. Am J Physiol 1988;255:R6–13.
23. Volpe M, Cuocolo A, Vecchione F, et al. Vagal mediation of the effects of atrial natriuretic factor on blood pressure and arterial baroreflexes in the rabbit. Circ Res 1987;60:747–55.
24. Volpe M, Odell G, Kleinert HD, et al. Effect of atrial natriuretic factor on blood pressure, renin, and aldosterone in Goldblatt hypertension. Hypertension 1985;7:I43–8.
25. Chartier L, Schiffrin E, Thibault G, et al. Atrial natriuretic factor inhibits the stimulation of aldosterone secretion by angiotensin II, ACTH and potassium in vitro and angiotensin II-induced steroidogenesis in vivo. Endocrinology 1984;115:2026–8.

26. Laragh JH. Atrial natriuretic hormone, the renin-aldosterone axis, and blood pressure-electrolyte homeostasis. N Engl J Med 1985;313:1330–40.

27. Wada A, Tsutamato T, Maeda Y, et al. Endogenous atrial natriuretic peptide inhibits endothelin-1 secretion in dogs with severe congestive heart failure. Am J Physiol 1996;270:H1819–24.

28. Rubattu S, Calvieri C, Pagliaro B, et al. Atrial natriuretic peptide and regulation of vascular function in hypertension and heart failure: implications for novel therapeutic strategies. J Hypertens 2013;31:1061–72.

29. Potter LR. Natriuretic peptide metabolism, clearance and degradation. FEBS J 2011;278:1808–17.

30. Heublein DM, Huntley BK, Boerrigter G, et al. Immunoreactivity and guanosine 3',5'-cyclic monophosphate activating actions of various molecular forms of human B-type natriuretic peptide. Hypertension 2007;49:1114–9.

31. Nishikimi T, Minamino N, Horii K, et al. Do commercially available assay kits for B-type natriuretic peptide measure Pro-BNP1-108, as well as BNP1-32? Hypertension 2007;50:e163 [author reply: e164].

32. Nishikimi T, Okamoto H, Nakamura M, et al. Direct immunochemiluminescent assay for proBNP and total BNP in human plasma proBNP and total BNP levels in normal and heart failure. PLoS One 2013;8:e53233.

33. Goetze JP, Hansen LH, Terzic D, et al. Atrial natriuretic peptides in plasma. Clin Chim Acta 2015;443:25–8.

34. Lee CY, Burnett JC Jr. Natriuretic peptides and therapeutic applications. Heart Fail Rev 2007;12:131–42.

35. Yandle TG, Richards AM, Nicholls MG, et al. Metabolic clearance rate and plasma half life of alpha-human atrial natriuretic peptide in man. Life Sci 1986;38:1827–33.

36. Morgenthaler NG, Struck J, Thomas B, et al. Immunoluminometric assay for the midregion of pro-atrial natriuretic peptide in human plasma. Clin Chem 2004;50:234–6.

37. Yancy CW, Jessup M, Bozkurt B, et al. American College of Cardiology F and American Heart Association Task Force on Practice G. 2013 ACCF/AHA guideline for the management of heart failure: a report of the American College of Cardiology Foundation/American Heart Association Task Force on Practice Guidelines. J Am Coll Cardiol 2013;62:e147–239.

38. Januzzi JL Jr, Camargo CA, Anwaruddin S, et al. The N-terminal Pro-BNP Investigation of Dyspnea in the Emergency Department (PRIDE) study. Am J Cardiol 2005;95:948–54.

39. Mueller C, Scholer A, Laule-Kilian K, et al. Use of B-type natriuretic peptide in the evaluation and management of acute dyspnea. N Engl J Med 2004;350:647–54.

40. Moe GW, Howlett J, Januzzi JL, et al, Canadian Multicenter Improved Management of Patients With Congestive Heart Failure (IMPROVE-CHF) Study Investigators. N-terminal pro-B-type natriuretic peptide testing improves the management of patients with suspected acute heart failure: primary results of the Canadian prospective randomized multicenter IMPROVE-CHF study. Circulation 2007;115:3103–10.

41. Maisel A, Mueller C, Nowak R, et al. Mid-region prohormone markers for diagnosis and prognosis in acute dyspnea: results from the BACH (Biomarkers in Acute Heart Failure) trial. J Am Coll Cardiol 2010;55:2062–76.

42. Dieplinger B, Gegenhuber A, Haltmayer M, et al. Evaluation of novel biomarkers for the diagnosis of acute destabilised heart failure in patients with shortness of breath. Heart 2009;95:1508–13.

43. Potocki M, Breidthardt T, Reichlin T, et al. Comparison of midregional pro-atrial natriuretic peptide with N-terminal pro-B-type natriuretic peptide in the diagnosis of heart failure. J Intern Med 2010;267:119–29.

44. Shah RV, Truong QA, Gaggin HK, et al. Mid-regional pro-atrial natriuretic peptide and pro-adrenomedullin testing for the diagnostic and prognostic evaluation of patients with acute dyspnoea. Eur Heart J 2012;33:2197–205.

45. Seronde MF, Gayat E, Logeart D, et al, Great network. Comparison of the diagnostic and prognostic values of B-type and atrial-type natriuretic peptides in acute heart failure. Int J Cardiol 2013;168:3404–11.

46. Berger R, Huelsman M, Strecker K, et al. B-type natriuretic peptide predicts sudden death in patients with chronic heart failure. Circulation 2002;105:2392–7.

47. Anand IS, Fisher LD, Chiang YT, et al. Changes in brain natriuretic peptide and norepinephrine over time and mortality and morbidity in the Valsartan Heart Failure Trial (Val-HeFT). Circulation 2003;107:1278–83.

48. Maisel A, Hollander JE, Guss D, et al, Rapid Emergency Department Heart Failure Outpatient Trial Investigators. Primary results of the Rapid Emergency Department Heart Failure Outpatient Trial (REDHOT). A multicenter study of B-type natriuretic peptide levels, emergency department decision making, and outcomes in patients presenting with shortness of breath. J Am Coll Cardiol 2004;44:1328–33.

49. Januzzi JL Jr, Sakhuja R, O'Donoghue M, et al. Utility of amino-terminal pro-brain natriuretic peptide testing for prediction of 1-year mortality in patients with dyspnea treated in the emergency department. Arch Intern Med 2006;166:315–20.

50. Doust JA, Pietrzak E, Dobson A, et al. How well does B-type natriuretic peptide predict death and cardiac events in patients with heart failure: systematic review. BMJ 2005;330:625.

51. Bettencourt P, Ferreira S, Azevedo A, et al. Preliminary data on the potential usefulness of B-type natriuretic peptide levels in predicting outcome after hospital discharge in patients with heart failure. Am J Med 2002;113:215–9.

52. Cheng V, Kazanagra R, Garcia A, et al. A rapid bedside test for B-type peptide predicts treatment outcomes in patients admitted for decompensated heart failure: a pilot study. J Am Coll Cardiol 2001; 37:386–91.

53. Fonarow GC, Peacock WF, Phillips CO, et al, ADHERE Scientific Advisory Committee and Investigators. Admission B-type natriuretic peptide levels and in-hospital mortality in acute decompensated heart failure. J Am Coll Cardiol 2007;49:1943–50.

54. Hsich EM, Grau-Sepulveda MV, Hernandez AF, et al. Relationship between sex, ejection fraction, and B-type natriuretic peptide levels in patients hospitalized with heart failure and associations with inhospital outcomes: findings from the Get with the Guideline-Heart Failure Registry. Am Heart J 2013; 166:1063–71.e3.

55. Wang TJ, Larson MG, Levy D, et al. Plasma natriuretic peptide levels and the risk of cardiovascular events and death. N Engl J Med 2004;350:655–63.

56. Gegenhuber A, Struck J, Dieplinger B, et al. Comparative evaluation of B-type natriuretic peptide, mid-regional pro-A-type natriuretic peptide, mid-regional pro-adrenomedullin, and copeptin to predict 1-year mortality in patients with acute destabilized heart failure. J Card Fail 2007;13:42–9.

57. Moertl D, Berger R, Struck J, et al. Comparison of midregional pro-atrial and B-type natriuretic peptides in chronic heart failure: influencing factors, detection of left ventricular systolic dysfunction, and prediction of death. J Am Coll Cardiol 2009; 53:1783–90.

58. Masson S, Latini R, Carbonieri E, et al. The predictive value of stable precursor fragments of vasoactive peptides in patients with chronic heart failure: data from the GISSI-heart failure (GISSI-HF) trial. Eur J Heart Fail 2010;12:338–47.

59. von Haehling S, Jankowska EA, Morgenthaler NG, et al. Comparison of midregional pro-atrial natriuretic peptide with N-terminal pro-B-type natriuretic peptide in predicting survival in patients with chronic heart failure. J Am Coll Cardiol 2007;50:1973–80.

60. Miller WL, Hartman KA, Grill DE, et al. Serial measurements of midregion proANP and copeptin in ambulatory patients with heart failure: incremental prognostic value of novel biomarkers in heart failure. Heart 2012;98:389–94.

61. Khan SQ, Dhillon O, Kelly D, et al. Plasma N-terminal B-type natriuretic peptide as an indicator of long-term survival after acute myocardial infarction: comparison with plasma midregional pro-atrial natriuretic peptide: the LAMP (Leicester Acute Myocardial Infarction Peptide) study. J Am Coll Cardiol 2008; 51:1857–64.

62. Sabatine MS, Morrow DA, de Lemos JA, et al. Evaluation of multiple biomarkers of cardiovascular stress for risk prediction and guiding medical therapy in patients with stable coronary disease. Circulation 2012;125:233–40.

63. Truong QA, Siegel E, Karakas M, et al. Relation of natriuretic peptides and midregional proadrenomedullin to cardiac chamber volumes by computed tomography in patients without heart failure: from the ROMICAT Trial. Clin Chem 2010;56:651–60.

64. Smith JG, Newton-Cheh C, Almgren P, et al. Assessment of conventional cardiovascular risk factors and multiple biomarkers for the prediction of incident heart failure and atrial fibrillation. J Am Coll Cardiol 2010;56:1712–9.

65. Barbato A, Sciarretta S, Marchitti S, et al, Olivetti Heart Study Research Group. Aminoterminal natriuretic peptides and cardiovascular risk in an Italian male adult cohort. Int J Cardiol 2011;152:245–6.

66. Maisel A, Xue Y, Greene SJ, et al. The potential role of natriuretic peptide-guided management for patients hospitalized for heart failure. J Card Fail 2015;21:233–9.

67. Kazanegra R, Cheng V, Garcia A, et al. A rapid test for B-type natriuretic peptide correlates with falling wedge pressures in patients treated for decompensated heart failure: a pilot study. J Card Fail 2001;7: 21–9.

68. Jourdain P, Jondeau G, Funck F, et al. Plasma brain natriuretic peptide-guided therapy to improve outcome in heart failure: the STARS-BNP Multicenter Study. J Am Coll Cardiol 2007;49:1733–9.

69. Lainchbury JG, Troughton RW, Strangman KM, et al. N-terminal pro-B-type natriuretic peptide-guided treatment for chronic heart failure: results from the BATTLESCARRED (NT-proBNP-Assisted Treatment To Lessen Serial Cardiac Readmissions and Death) trial. J Am Coll Cardiol 2009;55:53–60.

70. Pfisterer M, Buser P, Rickli H, et al. BNP-guided vs symptom-guided heart failure therapy: the Trial of Intensified vs Standard Medical Therapy in Elderly Patients with Congestive Heart Failure (TIME-CHF) randomized trial. JAMA 2009;301:383–92.

71. Troughton RW, Frampton CM, Brunner-La Rocca HP, et al. Effect of B-type natriuretic peptide-guided treatment of chronic heart failure on total mortality and hospitalization: an individual patient meta-analysis. Eur Heart J 2014;35:1559–67.

72. Arrigo M, Truong QA, Szymonifka J, et al. Midregional pro-atrial natriuretic peptide to predict

clinical course in heart failure patients undergoing cardiac resynchronization therapy. Europace 2017. [Epub ahead of print].

73. Redfield MM, Rodeheffor NJ, Jacobsen SJ, et al. Plasma brain natriuretic peptide concentration: impact of age and gender. J Am Coll Cardiol 2002; 40:976–82.

74. Wang TJ, Larson MG, Levy D, et al. Impact of age and sex on plasma natriuretic peptide levels in healthy adults. Am J Cardiol 2002;90:254–8.

75. McCullough PA, Duc P, Omland T, et al, Breathing Not Properly Multinational Study Investigators. B-type natriuretic peptide and renal function in the diagnosis of heart failure: an analysis from the Breathing Not Properly Multinational Study. Am J Kidney Dis 2003;41:571–9.

76. Wang TJ, Larson MG, Levy D, et al. Impact of obesity on plasma natriuretic peptide levels. Circulation 2004;109:594–600.

77. Mehra MR, Uber PA, Park MH, et al. Obesity and suppressed B-type natriuretic peptide levels in heart failure. J Am Coll Cardiol 2004;43:1590–5.

78. Daniels LB, Clopton P, Bhalla V, et al. How obesity affects the cut-points for B-type natriuretic peptide in the diagnosis of acute heart failure. Results from the Breathing Not Properly Multinational Study. Am Heart J 2006;151:999–1005.

79. Sarzani R, Dessi-Fulgheri P, Paci VM, et al. Expression of natriuretic peptide receptors in human adipose and other tissues. J Endocrinol Invest 1996;19:581–5.

80. Das SR, Drazner MH, Dries DL, et al. Impact of body mass and body composition on circulating levels of natriuretic peptides: results from the Dallas Heart Study. Circulation 2005;112:2163–8.

81. Daniels LB, Clopton P, Potocki M, et al. Influence of age, race, sex, and body mass index on interpretation of midregional pro atrial natriuretic peptide for the diagnosis of acute heart failure: results from the BACH multinational study. Eur J Heart Fail 2012;14:22–31.

82. Kube J, Ebner N, Jankowska EA, et al. The influence of confounders in the analysis of mid-regional pro-atrial natriuretic peptide in patients with chronic heart failure. Int J Cardiol 2016;219:84–91.

83. Chenevier-Gobeaux C, Guerin S, Andre S, et al. Mid-regional pro-atrial natriuretic peptide for the diagnosis of cardiac-related dyspnea according to renal function in the emergency department: a comparison with B-type natriuretic peptide (BNP) and N-terminal proBNP. Clin Chem 2010;56:1708–17.

84. McMurray JJ, Packer M, Desai AS, et al. Angiotensin-neprilysin inhibition versus enalapril in heart failure. N Engl J Med 2014;371:993–1004.

85. Mangiafico S, Costello-Boerrigter LC, Andersen IA, et al. Neutral endopeptidase inhibition and the natriuretic peptide system: an evolving strategy in cardiovascular therapeutics. Eur Heart J 2013;34:886–893c.

86. McKie PM, Burnett JC Jr. NT-proBNP: the gold standard biomarker in heart failure. J Am Coll Cardiol 2016;68:2437–9.

87. Gu J, Noe A, Chandra P, et al. Pharmacokinetics and pharmacodynamics of LCZ696, a novel dual-acting angiotensin receptor-neprilysin inhibitor (ARNi). J Clin Pharmacol 2010;50:401–14.

88. Schou M, Gustafsson F, Nielsen PH, et al. Unexplained week-to-week variation in BNP and NT-proBNP is low in chronic heart failure patients during steady state. Eur J Heart Fail 2007;9:68–74.

89. Fokkema MR, Herrmann Z, Muskiet FA, et al. Reference change values for brain natriuretic peptides revisited. Clin Chem 2006;52:1602–3.

90. Pankow K, Schwiebs A, Becker M, et al. Structural substrate conditions required for neutral endopeptidase-mediated natriuretic peptide degradation. J Mol Biol 2009;393:496–503.

91. Zile MR, Claggett BL, Prescott MF, et al. Prognostic implications of changes in N-terminal pro-B-type natriuretic peptide in patients with heart failure. J Am Coll Cardiol 2016;68:2425–36.

92. Solomon SD, Zile M, Pieske B, et al, Prospective comparison of ARNI with ARB on Management of Heart Failure with Preserved Ejection Fraction (PARAMOUNT) Investigators. The Angiotensin Receptor Neprilysin Inhibitor LCZ696 in Heart Failure with Preserved Ejection Fraction: a phase 2 double-blind randomised controlled trial. Lancet 2012;380:1387–95.

N-Terminal B-type Natriuretic Peptide in Heart Failure

Arthur Mark Richards, MBChB, MD, PhD, DSc[a,b,*]

KEYWORDS

- NT-proBNP • Heart failure • Diagnosis • Prognosis • Monitoring

KEY POINTS

- Amino-terminal pro–B-type natriuretic peptide (NT-proBNP) is an excellent rule out test in the dyspneic patient with suspected acute decompensated heart failure.
- Factors partially confounding of the test, especially in nonacute settings, include advancing age, preserved ejection fraction, renal dysfunction, obesity, and atrial fibrillation.
- NT-proBNP adds strong prognostic information at all grades of heart failure independent of standard clinical predictors.
- Serial measurement of NT-proBNP in chronic heart failure provides ongoing risk stratification and a guide to titration of treatment.
- NT-proBNP is the marker of choice in assessing possible acute decompensation and for serial monitoring in patients receiving combination angiotensin 2 type 1 receptor blockade-neprilysin inhibition therapy.

INTRODUCTION

B-Type natriuretic peptide was discovered in 1988.[1] Proof of the existence of amino-terminal pro–B-type natriuretic peptide (NT-proBNP) in the human circulation and its relationship to cardiac function were first reported by Hunt and colleagues[2,3] in 1995. The B-type natriuretic peptides (BNP) are predominantly synthesized and released constitutively from ventricular cardiac myocytes. A proportion of proBNP 108 is also stored in, and released (alongside atrial natriuretic peptide [ANP]) from, perinuclear granules in cardiac atrial myocytes. The prime stimulus for synthesis and release of BNP is myocyte stretch secondary to transmural distending pressure. On cleavage of proBNP 108; NT-proBNP 1–76 is released in a 1:1 ratio with its carboxy-terminal congener BNP 1-32 (**Fig. 1**). The biological actions of the cardiac natriuretic peptides (NP) indicate they constitute an endogenous compensatory system that acts to counter excess cardiac load and volume expansion. Actions include natriuresis, diuresis, vasodilation, and lusitropism, plus direct suppression of volume-retaining, vasoconstricting systems including the renin–angiotensin–aldosterone and sympathetic nervous systems. NP also have trophic actions opposing cardiac hypertrophy and fibrosis.[4] It is the relationship between intracardiac pressures and plasma concentrations of BNP and NT-proBNP that underpin their value as biomarkers in HF as now

Disclosure: The author received speaker's honoraria, advisory board fees and research grants from Roche Diagnostics, maker of the NT-proBNP immunoassay.
[a] Cardiovascular Research Institute, National University of Singapore, National University Heart Centre, 1E Kent Ridge Road, NUHS Tower Block 9th Floor (Cardiology), Singapore 129788, Singapore; [b] Christchurch Heart Institute, University of Otago, Riccarton Avenue, Christchurch 8014, New Zealand
* Cardiovascular Research Institute, National University of Singapore, National University Heart centre, 1E Kent Ridge Road, NUHS Tower Block 9th Floor (Cardiology), Singapore 129788, Singapore.
E-mail addresses: mdcarthu@nus.edu.sg; mark.richards@cdhb.health.nz

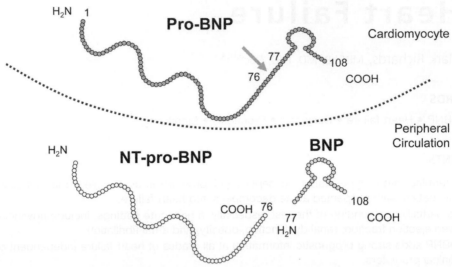

Fig. 1. Processing of pro–B-type natriuretic peptide (proBNP) to amino-terminal proBNP (NT-proBNP) and BNP. Alternative forms with cleavage by alternative dipeptidases: 3 to 32 (22%), 3 to 108 (60%). Commercial assays may not be specific for peptide (cross-react with other congeners or forms). BNP assay may measure 1-32, 3-32. Commercial assays validated for heart failure diagnosis, but may not reflect endogenous activity. (*Adapted from* Lam CS, Burnett JC Jr, Costello-Boerrigter L, et al. Alternate circulating pro-B-type natriuretic peptide and B-type natriuretic peptide forms in the general population. J Am Coll Cardiol. 2007;49(11):1193–202; with permission.)

mandated by authoritative international guidelines for the diagnosis and management of HF.

Amino-Terminal Pro–B-Type Natriuretic Peptide and Measures of Cardiac Structure and Function

Cardiac chamber wall stress, the prime driver of NP synthesis and release, in accord with the law of Laplace, is directly related to intrachamber pressure and chamber radius and inversely related to wall thickness. In concentrically hypertrophied hearts, as commonly observed in patients with HF with preserved ejection fraction (HFpEF), unit wall stress is less than in those patients with HF with reduced ejection fraction (HFrEF) and dilated left ventricles. Accordingly, plasma NP in acute decompensated HF (ADHF) are lower in HFpEF compared with HFrEF.[5,6]

NT-proBNP is correlated with several echocardiographic indicators of cardiac structure and function including:

- Left ventricular (LV) end-diastolic wall stress;
- LV ejection fraction (LVEF);
- E/e';
- LV longitudinal strain;
- LV circumferential strain;
- Left atrial dimensions;
- Right ventricular ejection fraction; and
- Right ventricular pressures.

Plasma NT-proBNP concentrations are related to a number of echocardiographically determined measures of cardiac structure and function in HF.[5–9] Iwanaga and colleagues[10] measured systolic and diastolic wall stress by echocardiography and cardiac catheterization, and related this key measurement to plasma concentrations of NP in patients with HF. A striking correlation between plasma BNP with end-diastolic wall stress ($r^2 = 0.887$; $P<.001$) seemed to be far stronger than the correlation with LV end-diastolic pressure ($r^2 = 0.296$; $P<.001$). NP levels seem to reflect LV wall stress more closely than other ventricular parameters in HF, and this relationship may better account for interindividual differences in plasma NP values than other measures.

Plasma NP concentrations reflect aspects of diastolic dysfunction independent of age, sex, renal function, body mass index, and LVEF. Plasma NT-proBNP (>600 pg/mL) and BNP (>100 pg/mL) are strong, albeit relatively nonspecific, independent predictors of restrictive filling the most severe grade diastolic dysfunction. In HF, plasma NT-proBNP correlates with E/e', a well-validated index of LV filling pressures, in addition to measures of LV compliance, myocardial relaxation, and left atrial dimensions. With respect to right heart function, plasma concentrations of B-type NPs are inversely related to right ventricular ejection fraction and directly related to right ventricular dimensions and estimated intraventricular pressures.[9]

An echocardiographic substudy of the phase II PARAMOUNT trial (LCZ696 Compared to Valsartan in Patients With Chronic Heart Failure and Preserved Left-ventricular Ejection Fraction) of valsartan-sacubitril therapy in HFpEF, demonstrated decreases in LV systolic longitudinal and circumferential strain that were significantly related to plasma NT-proBNP independent of age, sex, systolic and diastolic blood pressures, body mass index, LVEF, left atrial volume index, E/E', atrial fibrillation (AF), or renal function.[11]

Amino-Terminal Pro–B-Type Natriuretic Peptide in the Diagnosis of Acute Heart Failure

The relationship between cardiac structure and function and associated cardiac transmural distending pressures and myocyte stretch on the one hand with cardiac release and plasma concentrations of NT-proBNP on the other underpins the strength of NT-proBNP as a biomarker in HF. NT-proBNP has good diagnostic performance for discrimination of acute heart failure among patients presenting with new-onset dyspnea. Key publications include a report generated though data pooling from emergency department studies undertaken in New Zealand, the United States,

Spain, and the Netherlands.[12] The ICON study (International Collaboration on NT-proBNP) included data on 1256 patients presenting with new-onset shortness of breath. ICON data defined the sensitivity, specificity, negative predictive value, positive predictive value, and overall accuracy of NT-proBNP for the diagnosis of acute HF in acutely symptomatic patients, and these data have informed international guidelines for the diagnosis and management of heart failure.[13,14] Plasma NT-proBNP of 300 pg/mL acts as an excellent rule-out threshold with a sensitivity for ADHF consistently greater than 90%. A plasma NT-proBNP of less than this threshold indicates symptoms are highly unlikely to be due to acute heart failure. Acutely symptomatic patients with a NT-proBNP of less than 300 pg/mL are very unlikely to have acute heart failure. Specificity is improved by using age-specific cutpoints with 450, 900, and 1800 pg/mL performing well for age groups less than 50, 50 to 75, and greater than 75 years, respectively (**Table 1**).[12] The 2016 European Society of Cardiology guidelines for the diagnosis and management of heart failure strongly mandate measurement of NT-proBNP in the diagnostic workup for suspected acute heart failure emphasizing a rule out threshold of 300 pg/mL.[14]

Therapy with combined angiotensin 2 type1 receptor blockade and neprilysin inhibition (ARNI) has recently been shown to be superior to treatment with angiotensin-converting enzyme inhibition in chronic heart failure, offering an approximate 20% improvement in all key important clinical endpoints.[15] The new therapy has already entered authoritative guidelines and

Table 1
Optimal NT-proBNP cutpoints for the diagnosis or exclusion of acute heart failure among dyspneic patients

Category	Optimal Cutpoint (pg/mL)	Sensitivity (%)	Specificity (%)	PPV (%)	NPV (%)	Accuracy (%)
Exclusionary "rule out" cut point all patients (n = 1256)	300	99	60	77	99	83
Confirmatory ("rule-in") cutpoints						
<50 y (n = 184)	450	97	93	76	99	94
50–75 y (n = 537)	900	90	82	83	88	85
>75 y (n = 535)	1800	85	73	92	55	83
Rule-in, overall (n = 1256)	—	90	84	88	66	85

Abbreviations: NT-proBNP, amino-terminal pro–B-type natriuretic peptide; NPV, negative predictive value; PPV, positive predictive value.

From Januzzi JL, van Kimmenade R, Lainchbury J, et al. NT-proBNP testing for diagnosis and short-term prognosis in acute destabilized heart failure: an international pooled analysis of 1256 patients: the International Collaborative of NT-proBNP Study. Eur Heart J 2006;27:330–7; with permission.

its use is likely to become very widespread.[14,16] Neprilysin mediates cleavage of the biologically active carboxy terminals of ANP, BNP, and C-type NP, and prolongation of the circulating and tissue half-lives of these powerful effectors is presumed to underlie a significant proportion of the benefit offered by ARNI.[17] Accordingly, prescription of ARNI in chronic HF resulted in sustained elevations in plasma BNP, whereas NT-proBNP (which is not cleaved by neprilysin) decreased, reflecting impaired metabolism of carboxy terminal BNP and decreased cardiac release of NP, respectively (**Fig. 2**).[18] In this setting the relationship of NT-proBNP to intracardiac pressures and HF status, plasma is undistorted, whereas BNP is no longer a reliable marker. NT-proBNP but not BNP remains a valid marker during ARNI therapy. Where ARNI therapy is contemplated or already in place, NT-proBNP is the marker of choice in assessment of possible incident ADHF and for serial monitoring.

Amino-Terminal Pro–B-Type Natriuretic Peptide for the Diagnosis of Early Heart Failure in the Community

For the nonacute case with early or incipient decompensation, the much lower threshold of NT-proBNP of 125 pg/mL is recommended.[14] Diagnostic performance at this level in the nonacute setting is not as well-defined as it is for the case with severe acute symptoms. However, NT-

proBNP at about this level does aid in identification (area under the curve [AUC] > 0.9) of asymptomatic or minimally symptomatic LV dysfunction with an LVEF of less than 40% in community-dwelling patients as demonstrated by reports from the Olmsted County studies and from the ICON Primary Care study of approximately 5000 participants in an array of screening cohorts (**Fig. 3**).[19,20] NT-proBNP is also the only marker to have undergone a randomized, controlled trial to ascertain the additional diagnostic benefit it confers for the diagnosis of HF in primary care.[21] In a study of 305 patients assessed by 92 family doctors for suspected incipient heart failure (on the basis of exertional dyspnea and/or peripheral edema), the addition of plasma NT-proBNP measurements to clinical history and examination, significantly improved diagnostic accuracy by 10 patients per 100 assessed.

Modifiers of the Diagnostic Performance of Amino-Terminal Pro–B-Type Natriuretic Peptide

The typical elevation of plasma NT-proBNP in the setting of severe symptomatic ADHF is so pronounced (median values are >5000 pg/mL and are typically >40-fold greater than the levels observed in controls without HF) that this marker achieves an excellent "signal-to-noise ratio" for ADHF.[12] However, elevation of plasma NT-proBNP is not specific for ADHF. AF, renal failure,

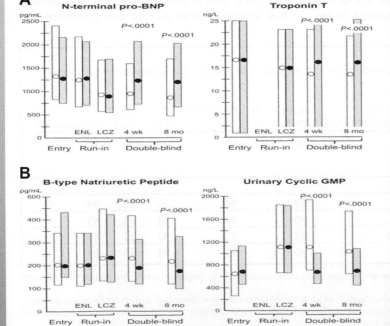

Fig. 2. (A) Median amino-terminal pro–B-type natriuretic peptide (NT-pro-BNP) and troponin T at entry and during single-blind run-in and double-blind periods. Medians are shown in circles, and 25%–75% interquartile ranges are shown in bars, where patients in the LCZ696 group are shown in white circles and bars and patients in the enalapril group are shown in black circles and bars. (B) Median values for BNP and urinary cyclic GMP according to same format as in (A). ENL, end of the enalapril phase of the run-in period; LCZ, end of the LCZ696 phase of the run-in period. P values give significance of difference between the 2 treatment groups. (From Packer M, McMurray JJ, Desai AS, et al. Angiotensin receptor neprilysin inhibition compared with enalapril on the risk of clinical progression in surviving patients with heart failure. Circulation 2015;131:54–61; with permission.)

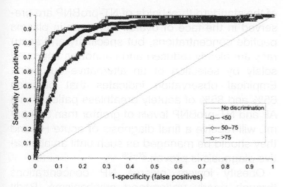

Fig. 3. Receiver operating characteristic curves for discrimination of a left ventricular ejection fraction of less than 40% among community dwelling asymptomatic or minimally symptomatic subjects according to age (<50, 50–75, and >75 years). (*From* Hildebrandt P, Collinson P, Fuat A, et al. Age-dependent values of N-terminal pro-B-type natriuretic peptide are superior to a single cut-point for ruling out suspected systolic dysfunction in primary care: the International Collaborative study of Natriuretic peptides in Primary Care (ICON-PC). Eur Heart J 2010;31(15);1881–9; with permission.)

pulmonary embolism, and a number of other causes increase NT-proBNP (**Box 1**). NT-proBNP level should be considered in concert with the clinical history, examination findings, and data from other tests, including a standard laboratory workup and cardiac imaging. Age, obesity, preserved ejection fraction, renal dysfunction, and AF may affect the diagnostic performance of NT-proBNP.

Consideration of confounding influences on NP plasma concentrations is necessary for interpretation of plasma NT-proBNP results in those with mild or early decompensated HF, or in epidemiologic settings where elevation of median plasma concentrations is not profound and background confounders become more intrusive.

Age is a strong determinant of NT-proBNP. This relationship is independent of kidney and cardiac function, and the exact underlying mechanisms remain unclear. Age-adjusted values enhance the specificity and accuracy of NT-proBNP in diagnosis of ADHF at the cost of some loss of sensitivity (**Fig. 4**; see **Table 1**).[12] An NT-proBNP level of 450 pg/mL or more in the presence of new onset dyspnea is highly discriminating for ADHF (AUC, 0.99) in those less than 50 years of age. Most HF patients are older and the AUC falls progressively to 0.93 and then 0.86 in patients aged 50 to 75 years (optimal threshold of 900 pg/mL) and those older than 75 years (1800 pg/mL), respectively. Age-adjusted values have been calculated for NT-proBNP but not BNP.[12]

Box 1
Causes of elevated plasma amino-terminal pro–B-type natriuretic peptide

Cardiac
- Heart failure, acute and chronic
- Acute coronary syndromes
- Atrial fibrillation
- Valvular heart disease
- Cardiomyopathies
- Myocarditis
- Cardioversion
- Left ventricular hypertrophy

Noncardiac
- Age
- Renal impairment
- Pulmonary embolism
- Pneumonia (severe)
- Obstructive sleep apnea
- Critical Illness
- Bacterial sepsis
- Severe burns
- Cancer chemotherapy
- Toxic and metabolic insults

LV structure and function influence plasma NT-proBNP. Specifically, plasma NT-proBNP plasma concentrations in HFpEF are approximately half those observed in HFrEF (**Table 2**) in both acute and chronic HF.[6,7,22] This reflects the integrated influence of ventricular internal dimensions, wall thickness, and intraventricular pressures (embodied in the law of Laplace) on unit wall stress and cardiomyocyte stretch, the primary driver of NP synthesis and release. In the event, the diagnostic performance of NT-proBNP in HFpEF is only marginally impaired in view of the high signal-to-noise ratio in acute HF, as discussed elsewhere in this article. In contrast, in the setting of incipient or treated HF, NP values often fall into the subdiagnostic range and this is particularly so in HFpEF.[23] This emphasizes the need to apply the recommended cutpoint values for acute HF in the appropriate setting; that is, with new onset of distressing breathlessness where acute HF is likely. When NPs fall into the "gray zone" between rule out and rule in values for acute HF (eg, NT-proBNP between 300 and 450 pg/mL <50 years of age; 300 and 900 pg/mL in those 50–75 years of age; and 300 and 1800 pg/mL in those >75 years of age), echocardiography is an invaluable diagnostic adjunct with

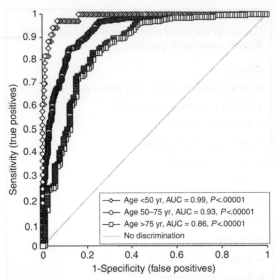

Fig. 4. Receiver operator characteristic curves for discrimination by amino-terminal pro–B-type natriuretic peptide of acute heart failure among dyspneic patients according to age. (*From* Januzzi JL, van Kimmenade R, Lainchbury J, et al. NT-proBNP testing for diagnosis and short-term prognosis in acute destabilized heart failure: an international pooled analysis of 1256 patients: the International Collaborative of NT-proBNP Study. Eur Heart J 2006;27(3):330–7; with permission.)

elevated E/e' and/or the presence of a restrictive filling pattern helping securing the diagnosis of HF.[24]

AF increases plasma NT-proBNP whether HF is present or not.[25–28] AF is a common complication of HF, and occurs in approximately 30% of populations with ADHF. AF reduces the discriminative performance NT-proBNP for newly symptomatic ADHF, reducing the AUC on receiver operator analysis to approximately 0.7, which is well below the approximately 0.9 observed in HF cases with preserved sinus rhythm (**Fig. 5**).[28] The sensitivity

of the standard thresholds of NT-proBNP are preserved in the face of overall increases in plasma peptide concentrations, but specificity and accuracy are clearly reduced and cannot be improved solely by selection of an alternative cut point. Empirical observation indicates that between 65% and 85% of acutely breathless patients with AF and NT-proBNP levels of greater than 300 pg/mL will receive a final diagnosis of acute HF and they should be managed as such until an alternative diagnosis is proven.[25–28]

Obesity lowers plasma NP concentrations through poorly understood mechanisms. Body mass index is actually inversely related to plasma NT-proBNP concentrations in both health and HF.[29–31] Unlike renal impairment or AF, which irretrievably impair the specificity and accuracy of plasma NT-proBNP, obesity shifts the optimal threshold but preserves discriminatory performance. The effect on the diagnostic performance of BNP at 100 pg/mL is pronounced, with a clear loss of sensitivity that has led to the recommendation to reduce the cutpoint to 50 pg/mL for those with a BMI greater than of 30 kg/m^2.[31] However, the test performance of age-specific thresholds of NT-proBNP seem to be less affected (**Fig. 6**).[30]

Plasma NT-proBNP increases as renal function decreases. Estimated glomerular filtration fraction rate are inversely related to plasma concentrations of BNP and NT-proBNP.[12,32,33] For BNP, this has led to the recommendation that the BNP threshold be increased to 200 pg/mL for an estimated glomerular filtration rate of less than 60 mL/min/1.73 m.[34] No specific corresponding change in cutpoint is generally applied to NT-proBNP values and the performance of age-specific NT-proBNP diagnostic thresholds seem to be less affected (**Table 3**).[34] The diagnostic specificity and accuracy of NT-proBNP are somewhat reduced in the presence of impaired renal function at any selected cutpoint.

Table 2
Median plasma concentrations of NT-proBNP in acute and chronic HFrEF and HFpEF

Category of Heart Failure	NT-proBNP Median (pg/mL)	N	Study/Trial	Ref
Acute decompensated heart failure				
HFrEF	6356	358	ICON	Januzzi et al,[12] 2006
HFpEF	3070	295	ICON	Januzzi et al,[12] 2006
Chronic heart failure				
HFrEF	895	3916	ValHeFT	Masson et al,[40] 2006
HFpEF	339	3480	I-PRESERVE	Komajda et al,[23] 2011

Abbreviations: HFpEF, heart failure with preserved left ventricular ejection fraction; HFrEF, heart failure with reduced left ventricular ejection fraction; NT-proBNP, amino-terminal pro–B-type natriuretic peptide.

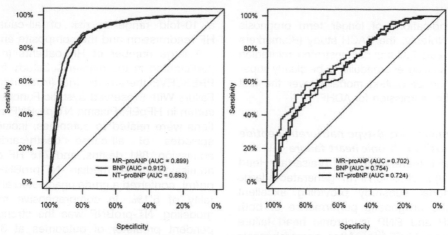

Fig. 5. Receiver operator curves for discrimination by amino-terminal pro–B-type natriuretic peptide (NT-proBNP; *blue*), BNP (*red*) or midregion amino terminal atrial natriuretic peptide (*blue*) of a diagnosis acute heart failure among breathless patients in (*left*) normal sinus rhythm or in (*right*) atrial fibrillation. (*From* Richards AM, Di Somma S, Mueller C, et al. Atrial fibrillation impairs the diagnostic performance of cardiac natriuretic peptides in dyspneic patients: results from the Biomarkers in Acute Heart Failure (BACH) Study. JACC Heart Fail 2013;1:192–9; with permission.)

Amino-Terminal Pro–B-Type Natriuretic Peptide and Prognosis in Heart Failure

Along with BNP and mid-region amino terminal pro-ANP, NT-proBNP is endorsed as an

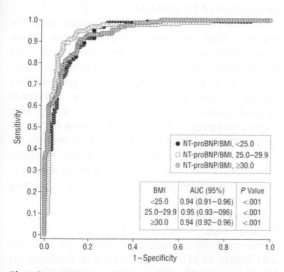

Fig. 6. Receiver operating characteristic curves for discrimination of acute heart failure amino-terminal pro–B-type natriuretic peptide (NT-proBNP) across 3 categories of body mass index (BMI; kg/m²). AUC, area under the curve. (*From* Bayes-Genis A, Barallat J, Richards AM. A test in context. neprilysin: function, inhibition and biomarker. J Am Coll Cardiol 2016;68:639–53; with permission; and *Data from* Bayes-Genis A, Lloyd-Jones DM, van Kimmenade RR, et al. Effect of body mass index on diagnostic and prognostic usefulness of amino-terminal pro-brain natriuretic peptide in patients with acute dyspnea. Arch Intern Med 2007;167(4):400–7.)

independent prognostic marker in acute and chronic HF and is endorsed for these indications in authoritative international guidelines on the diagnosis and management of HF.[13,14] Both single and serial measurements of NT-proBNP offer prognostic information in acute and chronic HF.[12,22,23,33,35–38]

Amino-terminal pro–B-type natriuretic peptide and early mortality in acute decompensated heart failure

The ICON study, although primarily aimed at assessing the diagnostic value of markers, also indicated NPs measured at admission for ADHF

Table 3
Impact of renal disease on the diagnosis of acute decompensated heart failure in patients presenting with dyspnea

	GFR (mL/min per 173 m²)	Area Under the Curve	Cutpoint (ng/L)
BNP	>90	0.91	70.7
	60–90	0.90	104.3
	30–59	0.81	201.2
	<30	0.86	225
NT-proBNP	≥60	0.95	900/450
	<60	0.88	1200

Abbreviations: BNP, B-type natriuretic peptide; GFR, glomerular filtration rate; NT-proBNP, amino-terminal pro–B-type natriuretic peptide.

From DeFilippi C, van Kimmenade RR, Pinto YM. Amino-terminal pro-B-type natriuretic peptide testing in renal disease. Am J Cardiol 2008;101:82–8; with permission.

provided indications of longer term prognosis (**Fig. 7**).[12] Notably, the BACH study (Biomarkers in Acute Heart Failure) demonstrated midregion amino terminal adrenomedullin to be clearly superior to NP in predicting mortality over the first 30 days after admission for ADHF.[39]

Amino-terminal pro–B-type natriuretic peptide and prognosis in chronic heart failure

The ValHeFT therapeutic trial (Valsartan Heart Failure Trial) in chronic HFrEF generated a large neurohormonal substudy providing excellent data on the prognostic performance of both NT-proBNP and BNP in chronic heart failure with reduced LVEF.[40,41] After comprehensive adjustment for demographic, biochemical, clinical, and imaging predictors, NT-proBNP remained an independent predictor of all-cause death and of readmission for HF. NT-proBNP performed more strongly than endothelin, aldosterone, or norepinephrine.[41] Median plasma NT-proBNP concentrations of 895 pg/mL corresponded with an unadjusted crude annual mortality of approximately 10.1%. Increments of 500 pg/mL in NT-proBNP conferred a 3.0% to 3.8% increment in risk of all-cause death or HF readmission. From first to tenth deciles of NT-proBNP, the ValHeFT population exhibited

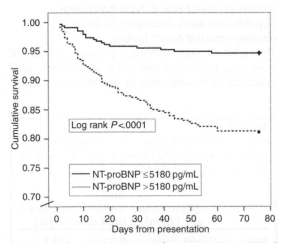

Fig. 7. Kaplan–Meier curves demonstrating survival rates of patients with acute heart failure (n = 720) during the first 76 days after presentation, expressed as a function of amino-terminal pro–B-type natriuretic peptide (NT-proBNP) concentration (log-rank test, P<.001). (*From* Januzzi JL, van Kimmenade R, Lainchbury J, et al. NT-proBNP testing for diagnosis and short-term prognosis in acute destabilized heart failure: an international pooled analysis of 1256 patients: the International Collaborative of NT-proBNP Study. Eur Heart J 2006;27:330–7; with permission.)

a 10-fold range in risk of all-cause death, HF readmission and the composite endpoint.

A large number of HF patients (n = 4128) participated in the marker substudy from the I-PRESERVE therapeutic trial (Irbesartan in Heart Failure With Preserved Systolic Function) of irbesartan in HFpEF. Plasma NT-proBNP concentrations were related to outcomes, including 1515 episodes of all-cause death/cardiovascular admission, 881 deaths, and 716 HF deaths/HF admissions.[23] A median NT-proBNP of 339 pg/mL conferred a crude unadjusted annual mortality of 5.1%. In comprehensive multivariate modeling, NT-proBNP was the strongest independent predictor of outcomes at 3 years of follow-up. Across septiles of NT-proBNP, risk extended over 7- to 20-fold ranges from 8.1% to 59.9% for the primary endpoint, 2.7% to 36.5% for death and 2.1% to 38.9% for HF death/HF admission. NT-proBNP, independent of multiple other accepted predictors, provided fine-grained prediction of clinical outcomes from low to very high risk. Findings from I-PRESERVE were also assessed by Anand and colleagues.[42] An additional report from I-PRESERVE displayed a 4- to 6-fold range of risk of these endpoints from the first to the fourth to quartiles of NT-proBNP.

Plasma NP criteria enrich trial populations for events, thus rendering sample sizes more manageable and providing greater certainty that the condition of interest, HF, is indeed present. The TOPCAT trial (Therapy for Adults with HFPEF) tested the efficacy of spironolactone in HFpEF in 3445 patients aged more than 50 years with signs and symptoms of HF and either a history of hospitalization with HF in the past 12 months or a NT-proBNP of greater than 360 pg/mL. Notably, outcomes were clearly improved by spironolactone in the subset of patients selected according to NT-proBNP.[43]

In the landmark PARADIGM trial (A Multicenter, Randomized, Double-blind, Parallel Group, Active-controlled Study to Evaluate the Efficacy and Safety of LCZ696 Compared to Enalapril on Morbidity and Mortality in Patients With Chronic Heart Failure and Reduced Ejection Fraction) comparing sacubitril and valsartan with enalapril in the treatment of HFrEF, plasma NT-proBNP was measured in a subgroup (n = 2080) of participants.[44] Those with baseline levels of greater than 1000 pg/mL (n = 1292) who achieved a decreases in NT-proBNP to less than 1000 pg/mL at 1 month (24%) after randomization incurred 59% fewer deaths or admissions with HF compared with patients with NT-proBNP remaining above this concentration (**Fig. 8**).

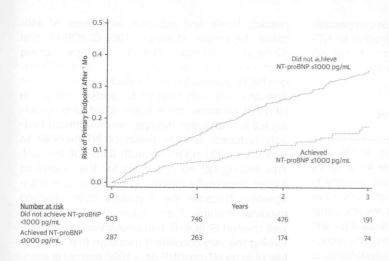

Fig. 8. Risk of primary endpoint after 1 month of randomization in patients with a baseline amino-terminal pro–B-type natriuretic peptide (NT-proBNP) of greater than 1000 pg/mL. The risk at 3 years of follow-up was 50% less in those who achieved an NT-proBNP of less than 1000 pg/mL than in those who did not. (*From* Zile MR, Claggert BL, Prescott MF, et al. Prognostic implications of changes in N-terminal pro-B-type natriuretic peptide in patients with heart failure. J Am Coll Cardiol 2016;68:2425–36; with permission.)

Markers to Replace or to Complement Amino-Terminal Pro–B-Type Natriuretic Peptide

Myriad additional candidate markers for HF have been reported. These include galectin 3, midregion proadrenomedullin, GDF 15, and ST-2.[45–47] NT-proBNP may combine with other markers including ST2, GDF15, galectin 3, midregion amino terminal adrenomedullin, and others to further refine risk stratification. Some are recommended within clinical guidelines as markers providing additional prognostic information in acute and chronic HF.[13,14] Many offer refinement of risk stratification when combined with NT-proBNP (**Fig. 9**).[14,45,46]

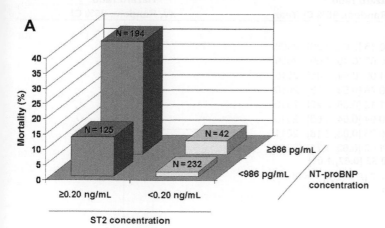

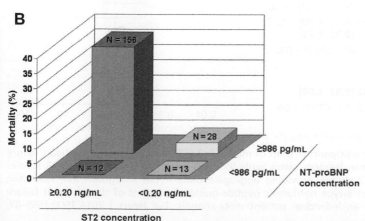

Fig. 9. Mortality rates at 1 year as a function of ST2 and amino-terminal pro-brain natriuretic peptide (NT-proBNP) concentrations among (*A*) all patients with dyspnea (n = 593) and in (*B*) the subgroup with acute heart failure (n = 208). (*From* Januzzi JL, Peacock WF, Maisel AS, et al. Measurement of the interleukin family member ST2 in patients with acute dyspnea: results from the PRIDE (Pro-Brain Natriuretic Peptide Investigation of Dyspnea in the Emergency Department) study. J Am Coll Cardiol 2007;50:607–13; with permission.)

Although a number of markers provide comparable or complementary prognostic information to NT-proBNP, at our present state of knowledge, no marker is superior to NT-proBNP in the diagnosis of HF.

Marker-Guided Therapy in Chronic Heart Failure

The associations between plasma BNPs and prognosis has provided the rationale for a series of controlled trials of hormone-guided therapy in chronic HF.[35–38] Although individual trials have variously yielded positive or neutral results, serial metaanalyses have consistently indicated benefit from guided therapy with greater than 20% reductions in total mortality and HF hospitalizations (**Fig. 10**)[37,38] Metaanalyses of trials of NT-proBNP–guided therapy in chronic heart failure suggest improved outcomes and confirm achievement of NT-proBNP of less than 1000 pg/mL confers a better prognosis. All trials of marker-guided therapy have consistently confirmed the strong association between achieved plasma B-type

peptide levels and outcome regardless of allocated treatment strategy. The GUIDE-IT trial (Guiding Evidence Based Therapy Using Biomarker Intensified Treatment) (ClinicalTrials.gov NCT01685840) was intended to provide definitive answers with respect to guided therapy in HFrEF.[48] However, it has been halted early reflecting full and effective therapy, which unprecedentedly reduced average levels of NT-proBNP to less than 1000 pg/mL in both limbs of the trial. This finding left no possibility for the marker to trigger meaningful intergroup differences in management because the 2 groups both received maximal therapy. Event rates were low in the well-treated GUIDE-IT trial population, again reinforcing the very consistent message that attaining low plasma NT-proBNP (ie, <1000 pg/mL) is associated with improved outcomes.

Biomarkers and Heart Failure Risk Scores

Although guidelines recommend the use of risk calculators to inform management decisions on advanced therapies such as ventricular assist

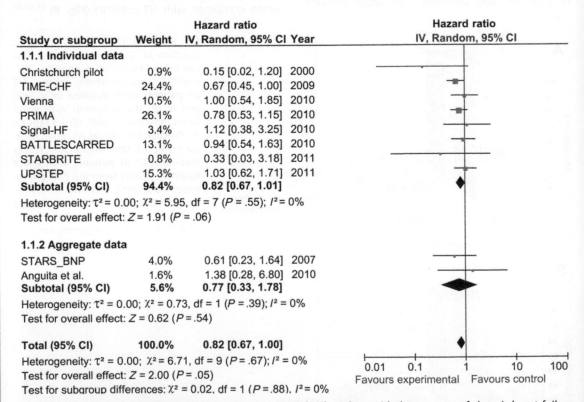

Study or subgroup	Weight	Hazard ratio IV, Random, 95% CI	Year
1.1.1 Individual data			
Christchurch pilot	0.9%	0.15 [0.02, 1.20]	2000
TIME-CHF	24.4%	0.67 [0.45, 1.00]	2009
Vienna	10.5%	1.00 [0.54, 1.85]	2010
PRIMA	26.1%	0.78 [0.53, 1.15]	2010
Signal-HF	3.4%	1.12 [0.38, 3.25]	2010
BATTLESCARRED	13.1%	0.94 [0.54, 1.63]	2010
STARBRITE	0.8%	0.33 [0.03, 3.18]	2011
UPSTEP	15.3%	1.03 [0.62, 1.71]	2011
Subtotal (95% CI)	**94.4%**	**0.82 [0.67, 1.01]**	

Heterogeneity: τ^2 = 0.00; χ^2 = 5.95, df = 7 (P = .55); I^2 = 0%
Test for overall effect: Z = 1.91 (P = .06)

1.1.2 Aggregate data			
STARS_BNP	4.0%	0.61 [0.23, 1.64]	2007
Anguita et al.	1.6%	1.38 [0.28, 6.80]	2010
Subtotal (95% CI)	**5.6%**	**0.77 [0.33, 1.78]**	

Heterogeneity: τ^2 = 0.00; χ^2 = 0.73, df = 1 (P = .39); I^2 = 0%
Test for overall effect: Z = 0.62 (P = .54)

Total (95% CI)	**100.0%**	**0.82 [0.67, 1.00]**	

Heterogeneity: τ^2 = 0.00; χ^2 = 6.71, df = 9 (P = .67); I^2 = 0%
Test for overall effect: Z = 2.00 (P = .05)
Test for subgroup differences: χ^2 = 0.02, df = 1 (P = .88), I^2 = 0%

0.01   0.1   1   10   100
Favours experimental   Favours control

Fig. 10. Forest plot of mortality among participants in trials of marker-guided treatment of chronic heart failure showing unadjusted individual and mean hazards ratios with 95% confidence intervals (CIs) for 8 studies providing individual patient data and 2 studies providing aggregate data. (*From* Troughton RW, Frampton CM, Brunner-La Rocca HP, et al. Effect of B-type natriuretic peptide-guided treatment of chronic heart failure on total mortality and hospitalization: an individual patient meta-analysis. Eur Heart J 2014;35(3):1559–67; with permission.)

devices and cardiac transplantation, the performance of such risk engines in individual patient management has been challenged.[14,49]

Risk calculators would likely be improved by incorporation of markers such as NT-proBNP. May and colleagues[50] assessed the performance of the Seattle Heart Failure Model in ambulant chronic heart failure and found, in a subgroup of 544 out of 4077 registered patients with BNP results available, that the marker modestly augmented the *c*-statistic for prediction of the composite endpoint of survival free from death, transplantation, or LV assist device implantation from 0.73 to 0.78 for events at 1 year. In the CORONA trial (Controlled Rosuvastatin Multinational Trial in Heart Failure) of rosuvastatin in HF, Wedel and colleagues[51] reported the *c*-statistic for prediction of all-cause mortality improved from 0.667 to 0.719 when NT-proBNP and high-sensitivity C-reactive protein were added to a clinical model. For predicting death specifically owing to heart failure, the *c*-statistic increased from 0.742 to 0.800.

SUMMARY

Plasma NT-proBNP is a powerful marker in heart failure. Its usefulness is best proven as an adjunctive rule-out test in the diagnosis of acute heart failure among patients with new-onset dyspnea. Guidelines recommend NT-proBNP be measured in all acutely symptomatic patients in whom the differential diagnosis includes acute heart failure. It is also a useful screening tool in the nonacute and primary care settings for identification of incipient HF and asymptomatic LV dysfunction (LVEF < 40%). Plasma NT-proBNP results are affected by age, preserved ejection fraction, renal dysfunction, obesity, and AF. Although these factors have little impact on the sensitivity and negative predictive value of B-NT-proBNP in the acute setting, they may reduce specificity and overall accuracy of the test and certainly require consideration when the test is turned to nonacute settings and use as an epidemiologic tool. NT-proBNP adds prognostic information at all stages of acute and chronic heart failure with a more than 10-fold gradation of risk of key adverse outcomes from first to tenth decile of plasma NT-proBNP concentrations. Serial measurements provide a tool to monitor HF status and prognosis and to facilitate titration of therapy. Achieving plasma NT-proBNP concentrations of less than 1000 pg/mL is associated with lower rates of death and hospital readmission. A range of more recently discovered markers rival NT-proBNP as indicators of prognosis, but none outperform NT-proBNP as diagnostic test. Risk stratification can be refined by combining NT-proBNP with another marker and multimarker strategies may come into use when they can be shown to enhance management and outcomes. Current HF risk calculators incorporating a selection of acknowledged clinical predictors are not reliable in the prediction of key outcomes in individual patients and are likely to be improved by the incorporation of data on markers like NT-proBNP.

REFERENCES

1. Sudoh T, Kangawa K, Minamino N, et al. A new natriuretic peptide in porcine brain. Nature 1988; 332:78–81.
2. Hunt PJ, Yandle TG, Nicholls MG, et al. The amino-terminal portion of Pro-Brain natriuretic peptide (Pro-BNP) circulates in human plasma. Biochem Biophys Res Commun 1995;214:1175–83.
3. Hunt PJ, Richards AM, Nicholls MG, et al. Immunoreactive amino-terminal pro-brain natriuretic peptide (NT-PROBNP): a new marker of cardiac impairment. Clin Endocrinol 1997;47:287–96.
4. Espiner EA, Richards AM. Atrial natriuretic peptide. An important factor in sodium and blood pressure regulation. Lancet 1989;333:707–10.
5. Maisel AS, McCord J, Nowak RM, et al. Bedside B-type natriuretic peptide in the emergency diagnosis of heart failure with reduced or preserved ejection fraction results from the breathing not properly multinational study. J Am Coll Cardiol 2003;41:2010–7.
6. O'Donoghue M, Chen A, Baggish AI, et al. The effects of ejection fraction on N-terminal ProBNP and BNP levels in patients with acute CHF: analysis from the ProBNP investigation of dyspnea in the emergency department (PRIDE) study. J Card Fail 2005;11(Suppl 5):S9–14.
7. Anjan VY, Loftus TM, Burke MA, et al. Prevalence, clinical phenotype, and outcomes associated with normal B-type natriuretic peptide levels in heart failure with preserved ejection fraction. Am J Cardiol 2012;110:870–6.
8. Troughton RW, Prior DL, Pereira JJ, et al. Plasma BNP levels in systolic heart failure: the importance of left ventricular diastolic and right ventricular function. J Am Coll Cardiol 2004;43:416–22.
9. Troughton RW, Richards AM. B-type natriuretic peptides and echocardiographic measures of cardiac structure and function. JACC Cardiovasc Imaging 2009;2:216–25.
10. Iwanaga Y, Nishi I, Furuichi S, et al. B-type natriuretic peptide strongly reflects diastolic wall stress in patients with chronic heart failure comparison between systolic and diastolic heart failure. J Am Coll Cardiol 2006;47:742–8.

11. Kraigher-Krainer E, Shah AM, Gupta DK, et al. Impaired systolic function by strain imaging in heart failure with preserved ejection fraction. J Am Coll Cardiol 2014;63:447–56.

12. Januzzi JL, van Kimmenade R, Lainchbury J, et al. NT-proBNP testing for diagnosis and short-term prognosis in acute destabilized heart failure: an international pooled analysis of 1256 patients: the International Collaborative of NT-proBNP Study. Eur Heart J 2006;27:330–7.

13. Yancy CW, Jessup M, Bozkurt B, et al. 2013 ACCF/AHA guideline for the management of heart failure : a report of the American College of Cardiology Foundation/American Heart Association Task Force on Practice Guidelines. Circulation 2013; 128:e240–327.

14. Ponikowski P, Voors AA, Anker SD, et al, Authors/Task Force Members. 2016 ESC Guidelines for the diagnosis and treatment of acute and chronic heart failure: the task force for the diagnosis and treatment of acute and chronic heart failure of the European Society of Cardiology (ESC) Developed with the special contribution of the Heart Failure Association (HFA) of the ESC. Eur Heart J 2016;37(27): 2129–200.

15. McMurray JJV, Packer M, Desai AS, et al, for the PARADIGM-HF Investigators and Committees. Angiotensin–neprilysin inhibition versus enalapril in heart failure. N Engl J Med 2014;371:993–1004.

16. Yancy CW, Jessup M, Bozkurt B, et al. 2016 ACC/AHA/HFSA focused update on new pharmacological therapy for heart failure: an update of the 2013 ACCF/AHA guideline for the management of heart failure: a report of the American College of Cardiology/American Heart Association Task Force on Clinical Practice Guidelines and the Heart Failure Society of America. J Am Coll Cardiol 2016;68(13): 1476–88.

17. Bayes-Genis A, Barallat J, Richards AM. A test in context. Neprilysin: function, inhibition and biomarker. J Am Coll Cardiol 2016;68:639–53.

18. Packer M, McMurray JJ, Desai AS, et al, PARADIGM-HF Investigators and Coordinators. Angiotensin receptor neprilysin inhibition compared with enalapril on the risk of clinical progression in surviving patients with heart failure. Circulation 2015;131: 54–61.

19. Costello-Boerrigter LC, Boerrigter G, Redfield MM, et al. Amino-terminal pro-B-type natriuretic peptide and B-type natriuretic peptide in the general community: determinants and detection of left ventricular dysfunction. J Am Coll Cardiol 2006;47:345–53.

20. Hildebrandt P, Collinson P, Fuat A, et al. Age-dependent values of N-terminal pro-B-type natriuretic peptide are superior to a single cut-point for ruling out suspected systolic dysfunction in primary care: the International Collaborative study of Natriuretic peptides in Primary Care (ICON-PC). Eur Heart J 2010;31:1881–9.

21. Wright SP, Doughty RN, Pearl A, et al. Plasma amino-terminal brain natriuretic peptide and accuracy of heart failure diagnosis in primary care: a randomised controlled trial. J Am Coll Cardiol 2003;42:1793–800.

22. Richards AM, Januzzi JL, Troughton RW. Natriuretic peptides in heart failure with preserved ejection fraction. Heart Fail Clin 2014;10:453–70.

23. Komajda M, Carson PE, Hetzel S, et al. Factors associated with outcome in heart failure with preserved ejection fraction findings from the Irbesartan in heart failure with preserved ejection fraction study (I- PRESERVE). Circ Heart Fail 2011;4:27–35.

24. Whalley GA, Wright SP, Pearl A, et al. Prognostic role of echocardiography and brain natriuretic peptide in symptomatic breathless patients in the community. Eur Heart J 2008;29(4):509–16.

25. Silvet H, Youg-Xu Y, Walleigh D, et al. Brain natriuretic peptide is elevated in outpatients with atrial fibrillation. Am J Cardiol 2003;92:1124–7.

26. Knudsen CW, Omland T, Clopton P, et al. Impact of atrial fibrillation on the diagnostic performance of B-type natriuretic peptide concentration in dyspneic patients: an analysis from the breathing not properly multinational study. J Am Coll Cardiol 2005;46:838–44.

27. Morello A, Lloyd-Jones DM, Chae CU, et al. Association of atrial fibrillation and amino-terminal pro–brain natriuretic peptide concentrations in dyspneic subjects with and without acute heart failure: results from the ProBNP Investigation of Dyspnea in the Emergency Department (PRIDE) study. Am Heart J 2007;153:9027.

28. Richards AM, Di Somma S, Mueller C, et al. Atrial fibrillation impairs the diagnostic performance of cardiac natriuretic peptides in dyspneic patients: results from the biomarkers in acute heart failure (BACH) study. JACC Heart Fail 2013;1:192–9.

29. Daniels LB, Clopton P, Potocki M, et al. Influence of age, race, sex and body mass index on interpretation of MR-proANP for the diagnosis of acute heart: results from the BACH multinational study. Eur J Heart Fail 2012;14:22–31.

30. Bayes-Genis A, Lloyd-Jones DM, van Kimmenade RRJ, et al. Effect of body mass index on diagnostic and prognostic usefulness of amino-terminal pro-brain natriuretic peptide in patients with acute dyspnea. Arch Intern Med 2007;167: 400–7.

31. Daniels LB, Clopton P, Bhalla V, et al. How obesity affects the cut-points for B-type natriuretic peptide in the diagnosis of acute heart failure. Results from the Breathing Not Properly Multinational Study. Am Heart J 2006;151:999–1005.

32. Maisel AS, Krishnaswamy P, Nowak RM, et al. Rapid measurement of B-type natriuretic peptide in the emergency diagnosis of heart failure. N Engl J Med 2002;347:161–7.

33. Richards AM, Nicholls MG, Espiner EA, et al. Comparison of B-type natriuretic peptides for assessment of cardiac function and prognosis in stable ischemic heart disease. J Am Coll Cardiol 2006;47:52–60.

34. DeFilippi C, van Kimmenade RR, Pinto YM. Amino-terminal pro-B-type natriuretic peptide testing in renal disease. Am J Cardiol 2008;101:82–8.

35. Lainchbury JG, Troughton RW, Strangman KM, et al. N-terminal Pro–B-type natriuretic peptide-guided treatment for chronic heart failure results from the BATTLESCARRED (NT-proBNP–Assisted Treatment To Lessen Serial Cardiac Readmissions and Death) trial. J Am Coll Cardiol 2010;55:53–60.

36. Pfisterer M, Buser P, Rickli H, et al. (TIME-CHF) randomized trial elderly patients with congestive heart failure the trial of intensified vs standard medical therapy in BNP-guided vs symptom-guided heart failure therapy. JAMA 2009;301:383–92.

37. Savarese G, Trimarco B, Dellegrottaglie S, et al. Natriuretic peptide-guided therapy in chronic heart failure: a meta-analysis of 2,686 patients in 12 randomized trials. PLoS One 2013;8:58287.

38. Troughton RW, Frampton CM, Brunner-La Rocca H-P, et al. Effect of B-type natriuretic peptide-guided treatment of chronic heart failure on total mortality and hospitalization: an individual patient meta-analysis. Eur Heart J 2014;35:1559–67.

39. Maisel A, Mueller C, Nowak R, et al. Mid-region pro-hormone markers for diagnosis and prognosis in acute dyspnea results from the BACH (Biomarkers in Acute Heart Failure) trial. J Am Coll Cardiol 2010;55:2062–76.

40. Masson S, Latini R, Anand IS, et al. Direct comparison of B-type natriuretic peptide (BNP) and amino-terminal proBNP in a large population of patients with chronic and symptomatic heart failure: the Valsartan Heart Failure (Val-HeFT) Data. Clin Chem 2006;52:1528–38.

41. Latini R, Masson S, Anand I, et al. The comparative prognostic value of plasma neurohormones at baseline in patients with heart failure enrolled in Val-HeFT. Eur Heart J 2004;25:292–9.

42. Anand IS, Rector TS, Cleland JG, et al. Prognostic value of baseline plasma amino-terminal pro-brain Natriuretic peptide and its interactions with Irbesartan treatment effects in patients with heart failure and preserved ejection fraction: findings from the I-PRESERVE Trial. Circ Heart Fail 2011;4:569–77.

43. Pitt B, Pfeffer MA, Assmann SF, et al, for the TOPCAT Investigators. Spironolactone for heart failure with preserved ejection fraction. N Engl J Med 2014;370:1383–92.

44. Zile MR, Claggert BL, Prescott MF, et al. Prognostic implications of changes in N-Terminal Pro-B-Type Natriuretic peptide in patients with heart failure. J Am Coll Cardiol 2016;68:2425–36.

45. Ibrahim NE, Januzzi JL. Beyond natriuretic peptides for diagnosis and management of heart failure. Clin Chem 2017;63:211–22.

46. Januzzi JL, Peacock WF, Maisel AS, et al. Measurement of the Interleukin Family Member ST2 in patients with acute dyspnea: results from the PRIDE (Pro-Brain Natriuretic Peptide Investigation of Dyspnea in the Emergency Department) study. J Am Coll Cardiol 2007;50:607–13.

47. Kempf T, Wollert KC. Growth-differentiation factor-15 in heart failure. Heart Fail Clin 2009;5:537–47.

48. The Guiding Evidence Based Therapy Using Biomarker Intensified Treatment (GUIDE-IT) trial (ClinicalTrials.gov NCT01685840).

49. Allen LA, Matlock DD, Shetterly SM, et al. Use of risk models to predict death in the next year among individual ambulatory patients with heart failure. JAMA Cardiol 2017;2(4):435–41.

50. May HT, Horne BD, Levy WC, et al. Validation of the Seattle Heart Failure model in a community-based heart failure population and enhancement by adding B-Type Natriuretic Peptide. Am J Cardiol 2007;100:697–700.

51. Wedel H, McMurray JJ, Lindberg M, et al. Predictors of fatal and non-fatal outcomes in the Controlled Rosuvastatin Multinational Trial in Heart Failure (CORONA): incremental value of apolipoprotein A-1, high-sensitivity C-reactive peptide and N-terminal pro B-type natriuretic peptide. Eur J Heart Fail 2009;11:281–91.

Soluble ST2 in Heart Failure

Cian P. McCarthy, MB, BCh, BAO[a], James L. Januzzi Jr, MD[b,c],*

KEYWORDS

- ST2 • Novel cardiac biomarkers • Heart failure • Prognosis • Risk stratification

KEY POINTS

- Soluble ST2 concentrations are closely associated with left ventricular hypertrophy, fibrosis, and ventricular remodeling.
- An elevated soluble ST2 concentration (eg, >35 ng/mL) is a predictor of adverse clinical outcomes in both acute and chronic heart failure.
- Unlike the natriuretic peptides, soluble ST2 is less affected by age, renal function, and body mass index.
- Combining soluble ST2 with other cardiac biomarkers (eg, N-terminal pro b-type natriuretic peptide NT-proBNP) may improve prognostic ability of each marker.
- In patients with chronic heart failure, soluble ST2 may be used to guide therapeutic intervention, however, studies are warranted.

INTRODUCTION

Heart failure (HF) remains a major public health concern, with a prevalence of more than 5.8 million in the United States and more than 23 million worldwide.[1] With an aging population, an expanding arsenal of effective HF therapies, improved survival rates after myocardial infarction, and a growing incidence of cardiovascular (CV) risk factors among the general population, prevalence of HF continues to increase.[2] Despite advances in therapy and management, HF remains a significant source of mortality, with 1 in 8 deaths in the United States associated with the diagnosis.[3]

In an effort to reduce mortality rates and improve morbidity, accurate identification of disease severity and prognosis, leading in turn to appropriate treatment, is a crucial component of HF management. In this setting, the use of biomarkers in patients with HF has grown in recent years, the most notable of which are the natriuretic peptides B-type natriuretic peptide (BNP) and its amino-terminal cleavage fragment (NT-proBNP). Although of value, BNP and NT-proBNP provide only one view of the biologic landscape in a patient with HF, which has led to the need for development of other biomarkers providing "orthogonal" biological information to the NPs.[4] Among the most promising of numerous novel HF biomarker candidates is suppression of tumorigenicity 2 (ST2). Several studies in both acute and chronic HF cohorts have illustrated the prognostic potential of this biomarker, independently and additive

Disclosures: Dr J.L. Januzzi has received grant support from Siemens, Singulex, and Prevencio, consulting income from Roche Diagnostics, Critical Diagnostics, Sphingotec, Phillips, and Novartis, and participates in clinical endpoint committees/data safety monitoring boards for Pfizer, Novartis, Amgen, Janssen, and Boehringer Ingelheim. Dr J.L. Januzzi is supported in part by the Hutter Family Professorship in Cardiology. Dr C.P. McCarthy has nothing to disclose.
^a Department of Medicine, Massachusetts General Hospital, 55 Fruit Street, Boston, MA 02114, USA; ^b Division of Cardiology, Department of Medicine, Massachusetts General Hospital, 32 Fruit Street, Yawkey 5984, Boston, MA 02114, USA; ^c Baim Institute for Clinical Research, Cardiometabolic Trials, 930 Commonwealth Avenue, Boston, MA 02115, USA
* Corresponding author. Massachusetts General Hospital, 32 Fruit Street, Yawkey 5984, Boston, MA 02114.
E-mail address: jjanuzzi@partners.org

Heart Failure Clin 14 (2018) 41–48
http://dx.doi.org/10.1016/j.hfc.2017.08.005

to other biomarkers.[5–8] Such studies have not gone unnoticed, with the American College of Cardiology Foundation and American Heart Association taskforce providing a recommendation supporting measurement of soluble (s)ST2 for additive risk stratification in patients with acutely decompensated HF (class IIb, Level of Evidence: A) and in patients with chronic HF (class IIb, Level of Evidence: B).[9]

In this article, we examine the biology, analytical considerations, and role of soluble ST2 (sST2) measurement in both acute and chronic HF.

THE BIOLOGY OF SUPPRESSION OF TUMORIGENICITY 2

The biology of the ST2 system is complex, and its role in CV disease is not entirely elucidated. ST2 is a member of the Toll-like/interleukin (IL)-1 receptor superfamily. The ST2 gene, found on chromosome 2q12, is expressed in 4 isoforms, 2 of which include a transmembrane receptor (ST2 ligand, or ST2L) and a soluble, serum circulating receptor (sST2)[10]; alternative promoter splicing and 3′ processing of the same mRNA appears to be responsible for the production of sST2 and ST2L.

First identified in 1989 as an orphan receptor,[11] early studies revealed ST2 as an important mediator in inflammatory processes involving mast cells and type 2 CD4+ T-helper cells; ST2 was subsequently associated with various inflammatory disease entities, including asthma, pulmonary fibrosis, rheumatoid arthritis, collagen vascular diseases, and septic shock.[12–16] Subsequently, in 2002, Weinberg and colleagues[17] identified the expression of both sST2 and ST2L by mechanically stressed cardiomyocytes via an in vitro model.

The discovery of IL-33 as the receptor ligand of ST2 in 2005,[18] provided new insights into ST2 signaling, with IL-33 demonstrating antihypertrophic and antifibrotic effects on cardiomyocytes, transduced by ST2L.[19] Analysis of rat neonatal cardiomyocytes and cardiac fibroblasts revealed that the administration of the sST2 blocked the favorable antihypertrophic effects of IL-33 in a dose-dependent fashion, signifying that sST2 may serve as an adverse "decoy receptor" for circulating IL-33.[19] In a subsequent in vivo study by Seki and colleagues,[20] mice deficient in ST2 had a greater degree of myocyte hypertrophy and fibrosis and poorer fractional shortening than wild-type mice after 4 weeks of pressure overload induced by aortic banding. Although IL-33 salvaged the hypertrophic phenotype in wild-type mice, it was unable to do so in ST2 knockout mice, further illustrating that IL-33/ST2 signaling

protects against adverse cardiac remodeling in vivo.[20]

Beyond the role of the ST2 system in mediating myocardial strain, a role for ST2 in the development of vascular disease has also been implicated. In mice studies, IL-33 demonstrated a reduction in aortic atherosclerotic plaque formation, whereas conversely, sST2 resulted in significantly more aortic plaque burden compared with control mice.[21] Further to this, sST2 has been identified as a marker of arterial stiffness, and is predictive of incident systolic hypertension.[22,23] Thus, sST2 is best viewed as a cardiovascular stress hormone, playing a role in both cardiac and vascular remodeling.

The source(s) of circulating sST2 remain elusive. Although messenger ribonucleic acid expression of ST2 is found in stressed cardiomyocytes, in coronary sinus sampling studies, no transcardiac gradient has been detected, suggesting concentrations of circulating sST2 are in fact derived from extramyocardial sources, presumably the vasculature. More data are needed to better understand the exact source(s) of sST2 production.

SUPPRESSION OF TUMORIGENICITY 2 ANALYTICAL CONSIDERATIONS

Early CV studies evaluating sST2 used imprecise enzyme-linked immunosorbent assay (ELISA) formats. Although providing useful prognostic information in a research setting, such assays were limited by low sensitivity for concentrations of sST2 in healthy subjects, and typically suffered from poor analytical precision with high coefficients of variation. As a consequence, only elevated sST2 values could be detected with any degree of precision. Fortunately, a highly sensitive ELISA for sST2 was developed (Presage ST2), which has low imprecision (coefficient of variation <5%) even at very low analyte concentrations.[24] This is the only assay that should be used clinically.

When measured in a cohort of community-based patients free of prevalent structural heart disease, expected/normal values for sST2 as measured with the Presage assay were generally higher in men, and were directly associated with age, prevalent diabetes, and hypertension.[25] Interestingly, sST2 values were not significantly affected by body mass index (BMI) or by renal impairment, a major limitation for BNP or NT-proBNP. An upper reference limit of 35 ng/mL was established for this assay; 95% of healthy subjects are below this threshold value. The Presage ST2 assay was approved by regulatory agencies both in Europe and the United States for prognostication in HF.

Although the Presage ELISA provides reliable measurement of sST2, lack of a more rapid format for sST2 measurement remained a limitation. Recently, a rapid quantitative lateral flow immunoassay for measurement of sST2 in human plasma has been developed, allowing for point-of-care testing. Although the Aspect-PLUS ST2 (Critical Diagnostics, San Diego, CA, USA) test has received regulatory approval Europe, it has yet to be approved by the Food and Drug Administration in the United States.

SUPPRESSION OF TUMORIGENICITY 2 AND ACUTE HEART FAILURE
Diagnostic Capabilities

The potential applications of sST2 in acute HF were assessed in the PRIDE (Pro-Brain Natriuretic Peptide Investigation of Dyspnea in the Emergency Department) study.[5] sST2 was measured in 593 dyspneic patients with and without acute HF presenting to an urban emergency department.[5] Concentrations of ST2 (measured with a preclinical research use only ELISA) were significantly higher in those dyspneic patients judged to have acute HF (0.50 ng/mL, interquartile range [IQR] 0.27–1.22 ng/mL) versus those without (0.15 ng/mL, IQR 0.06–0.42 ng/mL; $P<.001$).[5] The optimal ST2 cutpoint was 0.20 ng/mL, producing an area under the curve (AUC) of 0.74 for the diagnosis of acute HF (95% confidence interval [CI] of 0.70–0.78; $P<.001$), inferior to that of NT-proBNP for diagnosis of acute HF.[5,26] The diagnostic ability of sST2 was also assessed by Henry-Okafor and colleagues[27] in a study of 295 patients presenting to the emergency department with signs or symptoms of acute HF syndrome and who met the modified Framingham criteria for acute HF syndrome. sST2 concentrations were higher in subjects with acute HF than in those without acute HF (0.23 ng/mL [IQR = 0.11, 0.41], versus 0.17 ng/mL [IQR = 0.08, 0.29], respectively).[27] Unadjusted analyses indicated sST2 was significantly associated with a diagnosis of acute HF ($P = .02$).[27] However, this finding did not hold up in adjusted analysis (odds ratio 1.21; 95% CI 0.83–1.76; $P = .33$). The AUC for sST2 was 0.62 (95% CI 0.56–0.69) after adjusting for history of aspirin and steroid use, age, gender, race, and BMI.[27] The reason for differences in specificity for acute HF is likely explained by the reason for elevated concentrations of ST2: although HF is an important cause of sST2 rise, other pathologic processes may lead to higher sST2 concentrations.[13,16,28–30]

Suppression of Tumorigenicity 2 and Cardiac Function and Structure

In the PRIDE study, 139 patients had a 2-dimensional echocardiography during index admission (median 45 hours after admission).[31] sST2 concentrations were associated with higher left ventricular (LV) end-systolic dimensions and volumes, lower LV ejection fraction, reduced right ventricular (RV) fractional area change ($P = .05$), higher RV systolic pressure ($P = .005$), and RV hypokinesis ($P<.001$).[31] In multivariate regression, independent predictors of ST2 included LV ejection fraction ($P = .05$) and LV dimensions ($P<.05$), RV systolic pressure ($P = .002$), NT-proBNP ($P = .009$), heart rate ($P = .01$), and the presence of jugular venous distension ($P = .05$).[31] In a study by Rehman and colleagues[32] on 346 patients with acute HF, patients with preserved LV ejection fraction had lower ST2 concentrations (Wilcoxon rank-sum test: 0.37 [0.21–0.81] ng/mL vs 0.57 [0.30–1.1] ng/mL; $P<.001$). The investigators found no difference in ST2 concentrations among patients with HF due to ischemic versus nonischemic causes.[32]

Suppression of Tumorigenicity 2 and Prognosis in Acute Heart Failure

The utility of ST2 in clinical practice is best as a prognostic biomarker in HF (**Figs. 1** and **2**). This was initially established in the PRIDE study, where concentrations of sST2 were higher in patients who were dead at 1 year than in survivors ($P<.001$), with greater concentrations predicting substantial risk.[5] In multivariate regression analysis for predictors of death at 1 year, sST2 concentrations strongly predicted 1-year mortality in both patients with and without HF.[5] Similar results were seen in a study by Mueller and colleagues[7] among 137 patients with acute HF attending the emergency department of a tertiary care hospital. In this study of the Presage ST2 assay, median baseline sST2 plasma concentration was significantly higher in the patients who died than in those who survived (870 vs 342 ng/L, $P<.001$).[7] Kaplan-Meier curve analyses demonstrated that the risk ratios for mortality were 2.45 (95% CI 0.88–6.31; $P = .086$) and 6.63 (95% CI 2.55–10.89; $P<.001$) in the second tercile (sST2, 300–700 ng/L; 11 deaths vs 34 survivors) and third tercile (sST2 > 700 ng/L; 25 deaths vs 21 survivors) of sST2 plasma concentrations compared with the first tercile (sST2 ≤ 300 ng/L; 5 deaths vs 41 survivors).[7] In multivariable Cox proportional-hazards regression analyses, an sST2 plasma concentration in the upper tercile was a strong and independent predictor of all-cause mortality.

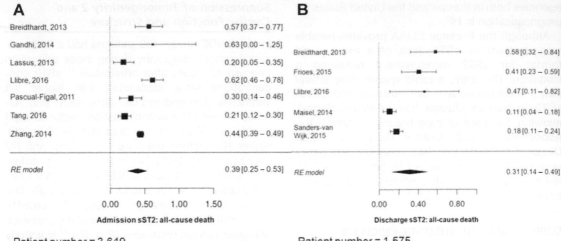

Patient number = 3,649
Event number = 729

Patient number = 1,575
Event number = 326

Fig. 1. Soluble ST2 and risk of all-cause death in acute heart failure. Admission (*A*) and Discharge Soluble Suppression of tumorigenicity–2 (*B*) forest-plot analysis. HRs and the corresponding 95% CIs are reported. Log10 values are provided (0 = no prognostic value). RE, random effects. (*From* Aimo A, Vergaro G, Ripoli A, et al. Meta-analysis of soluble suppression of tumorigenicity-2 and prognosis in acute heart failure. JACC Heart Fail 2017;5:292; with permission.)

Serial Measurement of Suppression of Tumorigenicity 2 in Acute Heart Failure

The serial measurement of ST2 in acute HF was first assessed by Boisot and colleagues[33] with daily measurement of sST2 in patients with acute HF. Interestingly, the investigators noted a dynamic change in sST2 levels during admission, with concentrations of sST2 decreasing rapidly after entry to the hospital in those who had uncomplicated short-term follow-up; in contrast, those patients who died by 6 months had a significant rise after admission.[33] In a prospective study on 72 patients with acute HF, sST2 was measured on admission and on day 4 of hospital admission.[34] Between presentation and day 4, sST2 concentrations decreased from 62 ng/mL (IQR 38–105) to 44 ng/mL (IQR 26–72; $P<.001$).[34] Both sST2 concentrations at presentation (hazard ratio [HR] 1.011, 95% CI 1.005–1.016; $P<.001$) and on

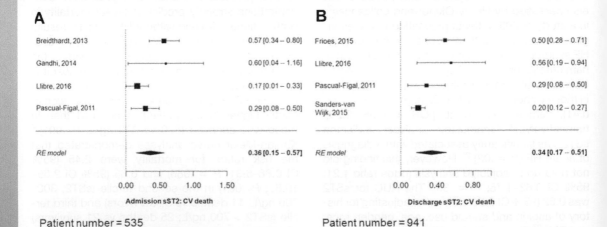

Patient number = 535
Event number = 98

Patient number = 941
Event number = 198

Fig. 2. Soluble ST2 and risk of cardiovascular death in acute heart failure. Admission (*A*) and Discharge Soluble Suppression of tumorigenicity–2 (*B*) forest-plot analysis. HRs and the corresponding 95% CIs are reported. Log10 values are provided (0 = no prognostic value). (*From* Aimo A, Vergaro G, Ripoli A, et al. Meta-analysis of soluble suppression of tumorigenicity-2 and prognosis in acute heart failure. JACC Heart Fail 2017;5:292; with permission.)

day 4 (HR 1.015, 95% CI 1.005–1.024; P = .003) were independent predictors of mortality.[34] Patients with sST2 ≤76 ng/mL at presentation and ≤46 ng/mL on day 4 had the lowest mortality rates (3%), whereas those with both sST2 values above these cutoff points had the highest mortality (50%).[34]

In another large study, serial sST2 measurements and prognosis was assessed in 858 subjects with acute HF enrolled in the ASCEND-HF (Acute Study of Clinical Effectiveness of Nesiritide in Decompensated Heart Failure) trial.[35] sST2 levels were measured in sequential baseline and during follow-up at 48 to 72 hours and 30 days. Higher sST2 concentrations were associated with increased death risk at 180 days (HR 2.21; follow-up HR: 2.64; both P<.001).[35] These results were not independent of covariates and NT-proBNP for baseline sST2 (HR 1.29, P = .243), but were borderline significant for follow-up sST2 (HR 1.61, P = .051).[35] Subjects with persistently high (>60 ng/mL) sST2 levels at follow-up had higher 180-day death rates than those with lower follow-up sST2 levels (adjusted HR 2.91, P = .004).[35] The results suggest that persistent elevation, as opposed to baseline measurement alone of sST2, has significant detrimental prognostic implications.

Combination with Other Biomarkers

The combination of ST2 with other CV biomarkers improves prognostication in acute HF. In the PRIDE study, the prognostic value of sST2 was additive to that of NT-proBNP, such that patients with elevations in both NT-proBNP and sST2 experienced the highest rate of mortality at 1 year, approaching 40%.[5] Similar results were seen in a prospective study of 195 patients with acute HF who had sST2 and BNP measured and were followed for 6 months.[36] There was a significant fourfold increase in risk of the endpoint for one elevated biomarker and sevenfold for both biomarkers elevated in HF reduced ejection fraction (HFrEF), and no association for one elevated biomarker and fivefold increase in risk for both biomarkers elevated in HF preserved ejection fraction (HFpEF).[36] Adding BNP to sST2 resulted in a net reclassification index of was 0.31 (P = .21) among patients with HFpEF and 0.70 (P<.001) among patients with HFrEF.[36]

Combining sST2 with high-sensitivity troponin T (hsTnT), and NT-proBNP levels, was assessed prospectively in 107 patients with acute HF.[37] Over a median follow-up period of 739 days, each biomarker was an independent predictor of mortality (sST2 per 10 ng/mL, HR 1.09, 95% CI

1.04–1.13; P<.001, hsTnT per 0.1 ng/mL, HR 1.16, 95% CI 1.09–1.24; P<.001, and NT-proBNP per 100 pg/mL, HR 1.01, 95% CI 1.003–1.01; P<.001).[37] Patients with all 3 biomarkers below their optimal cutoff at presentation were 0% mortality rates during follow-up, whereas there was a mortality rate of 53% among those with elevations of all 3 biomarkers. For each elevated marker (from 0 to 3), adjusted analysis resulted in a tripling of the risk of death (for each elevated marker, HR 2.64, 95% CI 1.63–4.28, P<.001).[37]

CHRONIC HEART FAILURE
Suppression of Tumorigenicity 2 and Prognosis in Chronic Heart Failure

In keeping with data in acute HF, studies of patients with chronic HF have demonstrated the prognostic ability of ST2 (**Figs. 3** and **4**). A recent meta-analysis affirms the importance of ST2 concentrations for prognostication in chronic HF; in this analysis of 7 trials with 6372 patients with chronic HF, sST2 had an HR of 1.75 (95% CI 1.37–2.22) for all-cause death and 1.79 (95% CI: 1.22–2.63) for CV death (both P<.001).[8]

Important findings may be gained from individual trials of sST2. For example, in a substudy of the Controlled Rosuvastatin Multinational Trial in Heart Failure (CORONA) study, Broch and colleagues[38] measured concentrations of sST2 in 1449 subjects with HF due to LV systolic dysfunction and measured a second level in 1309 subjects 3 months after randomization. During a median follow-up time of 2.6 years, after initial adjustment for established clinical and biochemical variables,

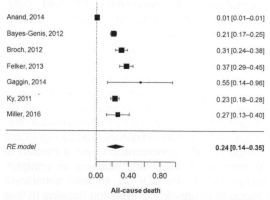

Fig. 3. Soluble ST2 and risk of all-cause death in chronic heart failure. Forest-plot analysis. HRs and the corresponding 95% CIs are reported. Log10 values are provided (0 = no prognostic value). RE, random effects. (*From* Aimo A, Vergaro G, Passino C, et al. Prognostic value of soluble suppression of tumorigenicity-2 in chronic heart failure: a meta-analysis. JACC Heart Fail 2017;5:284; with permission.)

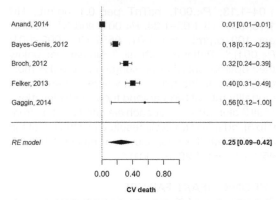

Anand, 2014   0.01 [0.01–0.01]

Bayes-Genis, 2012   0.18 [0.12–0.23]

Broch, 2012   0.32 [0.24–0.39]

Felker, 2013   0.40 [0.31–0.49]

Gaggin, 2014   0.56 [0.12–1.00]

RE model   0.25 [0.09–0.42]

0.00   0.40   0.80

CV death

Fig. 4. Soluble ST2 and risk of cardiovascular death in chronic heart failure. Forest-plot analysis. HRs and the corresponding 95% CIs are reported. Log10 values are provided (0 = no prognostic value). RE, random effects. (*From* Aimo A, Vergaro G, Passino C, et al. Prognostic value of soluble suppression of tumorigenicity-2 in chronic heart failure: a meta-analysis. JACC Heart Fail 2017;5:284; with permission.)

baseline sST2 was a significant predictor of all endpoints examined, including the primary end point of CV death, nonfatal myocardial infarction, or stroke, as well as death, and particularly worsening HF and hospitalization for HF.[38] Following the addition of NT-proBNP and C-reactive protein to the model, sST2 significantly predicted death from worsening HF (HR 1.57, 95% CI 1.05–2.34, P = .03), hospitalization for CV causes (HR 1.28, 95% CI 1.07–1.52, P = .006), and hospitalization for worsening HF (HR 1.30, 95% CI 1.04–1.62, P = .02).[38] Although most patients had no change in their sST2 serum concentration over the first 3 months, those who did had a reduced risk of hospitalization for worsening HF (HR 0.87, P = .02) and hospitalization for CV causes (HR 0.88, P = .006).[38]

As with acute HF, serial measurement of sST2 adds to baseline values in chronic HF. In a post hoc analysis of 151 patients with chronic HF due to LV systolic dysfunction, Gaggin and colleagues[39] performed serial measurement of sST2, NT-proBNP, HsTnT, and growth differentiation factor (GDF)-15. The investigators found a significant change in sST2 concentration over a median of 10 months of follow-up, whereas in contrast, neither hsTnT nor GDF-15 showed substantial change from baseline; correlating baseline to final values, a correlation coefficient of 0.67 was seen for sST2 compared with 0.87 and 0.86 for hsTnT and GDF-15, respectively.[39] In a Cox regression model for predicting cardiovascular events, a baseline sST2 level of less than 35 ng/mL was associated with a longer time to first CV event (HR 0.30, 95% CI 0.14–0.63, P = .002).[39]

Furthermore, a change in the sST2 status from less than 35 to at or above 35 ng/mL during the study was associated with significantly shorter time to first CV event (HR 3.64, 95% CI 1.37–9.67, P = .009).[39] sST2 results at 3 and 6 months added substantially to baseline concentrations for prognostication (P = .03 and P = .02, respectively).[39]

Beyond prediction of pump failure death, sST2 has also proven a predictor of sudden cardiac death (SCD) in patients with chronic HF. In a nested case-control study on 36 cases of SCD and 63 control patients (matched for age, sex, and LV ejection fraction) obtained from the MUSIC (MUerte Súbita en Insuficiencia Cardíaca) registry of patients with chronic HF (New York Heart Association functional class II to III, LV ejection fraction ≤ 45%), concentrations of sST2 were higher among patients who died (0.23 ng/mL [IQR 0.16–0.43 ng/mL] vs 0.12 ng/mL [IQR 0.06–0.23 ng/mL], P = .001) and were predictive of experiencing SCD (+0.1 ng/mL, odds ratio 1.39, 95% CI 1.09–1.78, P = .006).[6] In another study, serial changes in sST2 was found to be predictive of ventricular arrhythmia in a cohort of 684 patients enrolled in Multicenter Automated Defibrillator Implantation Trial (MADIT)-CRT.[40] Levels of sST2 were serially assessed at baseline and 1 year (n = 410). Although baseline concentrations of sST2 were not statistically associated with risk of ventricular arrhythmia (P = 0.21), in multivariable analyses (adjusting for randomization arm, age, gender, diabetes, left bundle branch block, LV ejection fraction, LV end-diastolic volume, renal function, baseline sST2, and BNP levels, as well as change in BNP), every 10% increase in sST2 resulted in a significantly increased risk of subsequent ventricular arrhythmia (HR [95% CI] = 1.10 [1.01–1.20]; P = .029) and death or ventricular arrhythmia (HR [95% CI] = 1.11 [1.04–1.20]; P = .004).[40]

Response to Therapy

A subanalysis by the PROTECT (pro-BNP Outpatient Tailored Chronic Heart Failure Therapy) group assessed the response of sST2 to medications. The investigators found the most substantial effect on sST2 was as a consequence of titration of beta blockers.[41] Interestingly, those with an elevated baseline sST2 concentration who achieved higher beta blocker doses (metoprolol succinate equivalent >50 mg/d) had substantially lower risk for CV events compared with those titrated to lower beta blocker dose, whereas in patients with lower sST2 concentrations at baseline, titration to higher dose beta blocker was associated with some reduction in risk, but a much smaller relative and absolute benefit.[41]

Similar results were seen in a subanalysis of the Valsartan Heart Failure Trial. Both baseline angiotensin-converting enzyme inhibitor and beta blockers were associated with lower sST2 concentrations, whereas digoxin and diuretics were associated with higher concentrations.[42] In that study, although there was a significant uptrend of sST2 values over time (+4.7 ng/mL per year) among placebo patients, treatment with valsartan significantly reduced this trend to a negligible 0.8 ng/mL per year.[42]

sST2 may also identify patients who benefit most from cardiac resynchronization therapy defibrillators (CRT-D). In a subanalysis of the MADIT study, patients with lower sST2 levels had greater reduction in the risk of death or HF with CRT-D than subjects with higher sST2 ($P = .006$).[40]

SUMMARY

sST2 is robust, prognostic biomarker in acute and chronic HF and is guideline-supported for risk assessment in these settings. Unlike the natriuretic peptides, soluble ST2 is not as affected by age, renal function, or BMI. The combination of sST2 with other cardiac biomarkers including NT-proBNP can improve prognostication. Future studies should focus on timing and frequency of sST2 testing and explore the utility of the CV biomarker to inform therapeutic decision-making in both acute and chronic HF.

REFERENCES

1. Roger VL. Epidemiology of heart failure. Circ Res 2013;113:646–59.
2. Bui AL, Horwich TB, Fonarow GC. Epidemiology and risk profile of heart failure. Nat Rev Cardiol 2011;8: 30–41.
3. Lloyd-Jones D, Adams RJ, Brown TM, et al. Heart disease and stroke statistics–2010 update: a report from the American Heart Association. Circulation 2010;121:e46–215.
4. Ibrahim NE, Januzzi JL. Beyond natriuretic peptides for diagnosis and management of heart failure. Clin Chem 2017;63:211–22.
5. Januzzi JL Jr, Peacock WF, Maisel AS, et al. Measurement of the interleukin family member ST2 in patients with acute dyspnea: results from the pride (pro-brain natriuretic peptide investigation of dyspnea in the emergency department) study. J Am Coll Cardiol 2007;50:607–13.
6. Pascual-Figal DA, Ordonez-Llanos J, Tornel PL, et al. Soluble ST2 for predicting sudden cardiac death in patients with chronic heart failure and left ventricular systolic dysfunction. J Am Coll Cardiol 2009;54:2174–9.
7. Mueller T, Dieplinger B, Gegenhuber A, et al. Increased plasma concentrations of soluble ST2 are predictive for 1-year mortality in patients with acute destabilized heart failure. Clin Chem 2008; 54:752–6.
8. Aimo A, Vergaro G, Passino C, et al. Prognostic value of soluble suppression of tumorigenicity-2 in chronic heart failure: a meta-analysis. JACC Heart Fail 2017;5:280–6.
9. Yancy CW, Jessup M, Bozkurt B, et al. 2013 ACCF/AHA guideline for the management of heart failure: a report of the American College of Cardiology Foundation/American Heart Association task force on practice guidelines. J Am Coll Cardiol 2013;62: e147–239.
10. Iwahana H, Yanagisawa K, Ito-Kosaka A, et al. Different promoter usage and multiple transcription initiation sites of the interleukin-1 receptor-related human ST2 gene in ut-7 and tm12 cells. Eur J Biochem 1999;264:397–406.
11. Tominaga S. A putative protein of a growth specific cdna from balb/c-3t3 cells is highly similar to the extracellular portion of mouse interleukin 1 receptor. FEBS Lett 1989;258:301–4.
12. Trajkovic V, Sweet MJ, Xu D. T1/ST2–an IL-1 receptor-like modulator of immune responses. Cytokine Growth Factor Rev 2004;15:87–95.
13. Oshikawa K, Kuroiwa K, Tago K, et al. Elevated soluble ST2 protein levels in sera of patients with asthma with an acute exacerbation. Am J Respir Crit Care Med 2001;164:277–81.
14. Leung BP, Xu D, Culshaw S, et al. A novel therapy of murine collagen-induced arthritis with soluble t1/ST2. J Immunol 2004;173:145–50.
15. Kuroiwa K, Arai T, Okazaki H, et al. Identification of human ST2 protein in the sera of patients with autoimmune diseases. Biochem Biophys Res Commun 2001;284:1104–8.
16. Brunner M, Krenn C, Roth G, et al. Increased levels of soluble ST2 protein and igg1 production in patients with sepsis and trauma. Intensive Care Med 2004;30:1468–73.
17. Weinberg EO, Shimpo M, De Keulenaer GW, et al. Expression and regulation of ST2, an interleukin-1 receptor family member, in cardiomyocytes and myocardial infarction. Circulation 2002;106:2961–6.
18. Schmitz J, Owyang A, Oldham E, et al. Il-33, an interleukin-1-like cytokine that signals via the il-1 receptor-related protein ST2 and induces T helper type 2-associated cytokines. Immunity 2005;23: 479–90.
19. Sanada S, Hakuno D, Higgins LJ, et al. IL-33 and ST2 comprise a critical biomechanically induced and cardioprotective signaling system. J Clin Invest 2007;117:1538–49.
20. Seki K, Sanada S, Kudinova AY, et al. Interleukin-33 prevents apoptosis and improves survival after

experimental myocardial infarction through ST2 signaling. Circ Heart Fail 2009;2:684–91.

21. Miller AM, Xu D, Asquith DL, et al. IL-33 reduces the development of atherosclerosis. J Exp Med 2008; 205:339–46.

22. Kim SH, Kim HL, Lim WH, et al. Soluble ST2 is a novel marker of aortic stiffness and arteriosclerosis measured by invasive hemodynamic study. Atherosclerosis 2016;252:e165.

23. Ho JE, Larson MG, Ghorbani A, et al. Soluble ST2 predicts elevated SBP in the community. J Hypertens 2013;31:1431–6.

24. Dieplinger B, Januzzi JL Jr, Steinmair M, et al. Analytical and clinical evaluation of a novel high-sensitivity assay for measurement of soluble ST2 in human plasma— the Presage™ ST2 assay. Clin Chim Acta 2009;409:33–40.

25. Coglianese EE, Larson MG, Vasan RS, et al. Distribution and clinical correlates of the interleukin receptor family member soluble ST2 in the Framingham Heart Study. Clin Chem 2012;58:1673–81.

26. Januzzi JL Jr, Camargo CA, Anwaruddin S, et al. The N-terminal pro-BNP investigation of dyspnea in the emergency department (pride) study. Am J Cardiol 2005;95:948–54.

27. Henry-Okafor Q, Collins SP, Jenkins CA, et al. Soluble ST2 as a diagnostic and prognostic marker for acute heart failure syndromes. Open Biomark J 2012;2012:1–8.

28. Brown AM, Wu AH, Clopton P, et al. ST2 in emergency department chest pain patients with potential acute coronary syndromes. Ann Emerg Med 2007; 50:153–8, 158.e1.

29. Martinez-Rumayor A, Camargo CA, Green SM, et al. Soluble ST2 plasma concentrations predict 1-year mortality in acutely dyspneic emergency department patients with pulmonary disease. Am J Clin Pathol 2008;130:578–84.

30. Bajwa EK, Volk JA, Christiani DC, et al. Prognostic and diagnostic value of plasma soluble ST2 concentrations in acute respiratory distress syndrome. Crit Care Med 2013;41:2521–31.

31. Shah RV, Chen-Tournoux AA, Picard MH, et al. Serum levels of the interleukin-1 receptor family member ST2, cardiac structure and function, and long-term mortality in patients with acute dyspnea. Circ Heart Fail 2009;2:311–9.

32. Rehman SU, Mueller T, Januzzi JL Jr. Characteristics of the novel interleukin family biomarker ST2 in patients with acute heart failure. J Am Coll Cardiol 2008;52:1458–65.

33. Boisot S, Beede J, Isakson S, et al. Serial sampling of ST2 predicts 90-day mortality following destabilized heart failure. J Card Fail 2008;14:732–8.

34. Manzano-Fernandez S, Januzzi JL, Pastor-Perez FJ, et al. Serial monitoring of soluble interleukin family member ST2 in patients with acutely decompensated heart failure. Cardiology 2012;122:158–66.

35. Tang WH, Wu Y, Grodin JL, et al. Prognostic value of baseline and changes in circulating soluble ST2 levels and the effects of nesiritide in acute decompensated heart failure. JACC Heart Fail 2016;4:68–77.

36. Frioes F, Lourenco P, Laszczynska O, et al. Prognostic value of sST2 added to BNP in acute heart failure with preserved or reduced ejection fraction. Clin Res Cardiol 2015;104:491–9.

37. Pascual-Figal DA, Manzano-Fernández S, Boronat M, et al. Soluble ST2, high-sensitivity troponin t- and N-terminal pro-b-type natriuretic peptide: complementary role for risk stratification in acutely decompensated heart failure. Eur J Heart Fail 2011;13: 718–25.

38. Broch K, Ueland T, Nymo SH, et al. Soluble ST2 is associated with adverse outcome in patients with heart failure of ischaemic aetiology. Eur J Heart Fail 2012;14:268–77.

39. Gaggin HK, Szymonifka J, Bhardwaj A, et al. Head-to-head comparison of serial soluble ST2, growth differentiation factor-15, and highly-sensitive troponin t measurements in patients with chronic heart failure. JACC Heart Fail 2014;2:65–72.

40. Skali H, Gerwien R, Meyer TE, et al. Soluble ST2 and risk of arrhythmias, heart failure, or death in patients with mildly symptomatic heart failure: results from MADIT-CRT. J Cardiovasc Transl Res 2016;9(5–6): 421–8.

41. Gaggin HK, Motiwala S, Bhardwaj A, et al. Soluble concentrations of the interleukin receptor family member ST2 and beta-blocker therapy in chronic heart failure. Circ Heart Fail 2013;6:1206–13.

42. Anand IS, Rector TS, Kuskowski M, et al. Prognostic value of soluble ST2 in the Valsartan Heart Failure Trial. Circ Heart Fail 2014;7:418–26.

Adrenomedullin as a Biomarker of Heart Failure

Toshio Nishikimi, MD, PhD[a,b,*],
Yasuaki Nakagawa, MD, PhD[a]

KEYWORDS

- Adrenomedullin • Heart failure • Mid-regional pro-adrenomedullin • B-type natriuretic peptide (BNP)

KEY POINTS

- Adrenomedullin (AM) assays and absolute plasma AM levels in healthy subjects.
- Two molecular forms of AM: AM-mature and AM-glycine.
- Origin of plasma AM and its metabolic clearance.
- Plasma AM levels in heart failure.
- Plasma mid-regional pro-adrenomedullin levels as a prognostic indicator of heart failure.
- Pathophysiological significance of plasma AM in heart failure.

INTRODUCTION

A number of neurohumoral factors contribute to cardiovascular regulation and to the pathophysiology of heart failure.[1] Among these is adrenomedullin (AM), a potent, long-lasting, vasodilatory peptide originally discovered in the acid extract of human pheochromocytoma tissue.[2] AM expression is widely distributed in the cardiovascular system, including the heart, blood vessels, and kidneys.[3] In addition, AM and its receptor components, which include calcitonin receptor-like receptor and receptor activity modifying protein (RAMP)2 and RAMP3, colocalize in those regions, suggesting AM acts in an autocrine and/or paracrine fashion to exert its effects on cardiovascular function.[4] Those effects of AM include positive inotropy and inhibitory effects on cardiomyocyte hypertrophy and proliferation and collagen production in cardiac fibroblasts.[4] This suggests AM acts as an antifibrotic, antihypertrophic, and positive inotropic factor in the failing heart.[5] In addition, antiapoptotic, angiogenic, anti-inflammatory and antioxidant effects of AM have also been reported.[6] This suggests AM plays a protective role during heart failure. Indeed, acute administration of AM during experimental[7] and human heart failure[8] has been shown to exert beneficial vasodilatory, diuretic, natriuretic, and positive inotropic effects. Here, we review recent study results and describe the significance of AM as a biomarker in heart failure.

Adrenomedullin Assays and Absolute Plasma Adrenomedullin Levels in Healthy Subjects

AM is produced from its precursor in a 2-step enzymatic reaction.[6] First, the AM precursor

Disclosure Statement: There is no conflict of interest to disclose.
This study was supported in part by Scientific Research Grants-in-Aid 25126712, 15K09138 (to T. Nishikimi), and 16K09498 (to Y. Nakagawa) from the Ministry of Education, Culture, Sports, Science and Technology of Japan.
[a] Department of Cardiovascular Medicine, Graduate School of Medicine Kyoto University, 54, Shogoin-Kawara-cho, Sakyo-ku, Kyoto 606-8507, Japan; [b] Department of Medicine, Wakakusa-Tatsuma Rehabilitation Hospital, 1580 Tatsuma, Daito City, Osaka 574-0012, Japan
* Corresponding author. Department of Cardiovascular Medicine, Kyoto University Graduate School of Medicine, 54, Shogoin-Kawara-cho, Sakyo-ku, Kyoto 606-8507, Japan.
E-mail address: nishikim@kuhp.kyoto-u.ac.jp

composed of 185 amino acids is cleaved to glycine-extended AM (AM-glycine), a 53-amino acid peptide that is an inactive intermediate form of AM. This is followed by enzymatic amidation, which converts AM-glycine to active mature AM (AM-mature), a 52-amino acid peptide with a C-terminal amide structure (**Fig. 1**). Kitamura and colleagues[9] were the first to develop a radioimmunoassay system for AM after extracting the peptide from plasma. They reported plasma AM levels to be 3.3 fmol/mL in healthy subjects. Other investigators also developed their own radioimmunoassay using polyclonal antibodies and reported plasma AM levels to be 3 to 8 fmol/mL. These assay systems have been carefully validated using high-performance liquid chromatography to show that immunoreactive AM from human plasma co-elutes with authentic human AM.[10,11] Thus the absolute plasma levels of AM in normal human subjects consistently range between 1 and 10 fmol/mL. Recently, the MR-proAM assay was established. MR-proAM is inactive and stable with a half-life that is longer than that of AM. Plasma MR-proAM levels are approximately 20 to 30 times higher than plasma AM levels.[12] In general, sex and age do not affect plasma AM levels,

and no circadian variation in plasma AM levels has yet been detected in healthy humans.[13]

Two Molecular Forms of Adrenomedullin: Adrenomedullin-Mature and Adrenomedullin-glycine

Kitamura and colleagues[14] reported that 2 molecular forms of AM, AM-mature and AM-glycine, circulate in human blood and that the major molecular form in the circulation is AM-glycine. They measured AM-mature and AM-glycine levels using 2 radioimmunoassay systems after extraction of the peptides form large amounts of plasma.

Ohta and colleagues[15,16] developed immunoradiometric assay kits for the measurement of AM-mature and AM-total (AM-total = AM-mature + AM-glycine). Both kits use 2 monoclonal antibodies against human AM. In both kits, one antibody recognizes the ring structure of human AM. In addition, a second antibody recognizes the carboxy-terminal sequence in the AM-mature kit or AM (25–36) in the AM-total kit. The assay measures human AM-mature or AM-total by sandwiching the peptide between 2 antibodies without extraction of the plasma. Reverse-phase

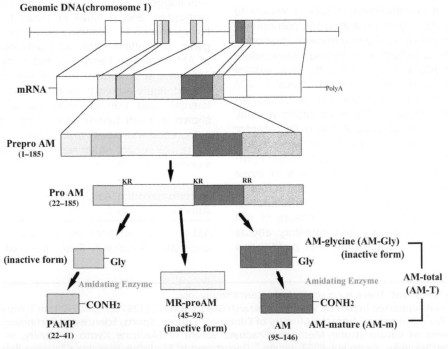

Fig. 1. Biosynthesis of AM. AM, pro-adrenomedullin N-terminal 20 peptide (PAMP) and mid-regional AM are synthesized from the same AM precursor (prepro AM: 185 amino acids). Removal of the signal peptide yields proAM. ProAM is then processed to glycine-extended AM (AM-Gly), glycine-extended PAMP and mid-regional AM. AM-Gly and glycine-extended PAMP are inactive intermediate forms of AM and PAMP. AM-Gly and glycine-extended PAMP are then converted to active mature AM (AM-m) and PAMP with a C-terminal amide structure through enzymatic amidation. AM-total = (AM-mature) + (AM-glycine).

high-performance liquid chromatography revealed that the major peak of immunoreactive AM detected with the immunoradiometric assay kits for both AM-mature and AM-total was identical to synthetic human AM (1–52). Using these kits, we and others reported that levels of AM-total in normal human plasma are approximately 10 fmol/mL.[17] In hypertension, renal failure, congestive heart failure, acute myocardial infarction, and pulmonary hypertension, plasma levels of both AM-total and AM-mature levels are increased, but the ratio of AM-total to AM-mature does not change significantly.[13,18,19]

When we used the 2-antibody system to measure AM-mature and AM-total in rat tissue and plasma, we found that the major molecular form in plasma is AM-glycine, as is the case in human plasma.[20] However, the major molecular AM form is AM-mature in left ventricular tissue from both normotensive and hypertensive rats, and the AM-mature/AM-total ratio is further increased in cases of severe left ventricular hypertrophy.[21,22] This means that AM-mature acts mainly as an autocrine/paracrine factor and is metabolized within the tissue. On the other hand, because AM-glycine does not bind to the receptors in the tissue, the AM-mature/AM-glycine ratio is higher in tissue than in plasma.

Origin of Plasma Adrenomedullin and Its Metabolic Clearance

AM was initially discovered in human pheochromocytoma by monitoring cAMP activity in rat platelets.[1] AM mRNA is highly expressed not only in pheochromocytoma, but also in the normal adrenal medulla and in kidneys, lungs, and cardiac ventricles.[2] But whether these organs secrete AM into the circulation was not initially fully understood. To investigate the sites of production and clearance of AM in humans, we collected samples of both arterial and venous blood across the adrenal gland, kidney, lung, and heart, and measured plasma AM levels using a radioimmunoassay.[23] We detected no step-up of plasma AM levels in the coronary sinus, renal vein, or adrenal vein. Moreover, there were no significant differences in plasma AM levels among several sites on the right side of the heart, including the inferior portion of the inferior vena cava, superior portion of the inferior vena cava, superior vena cava, right atrium, right ventricle, and pulmonary artery. Plasma AM levels in the aorta were slightly but significantly lower than in the pulmonary artery. Furthermore, in a patient with a pheochromocytoma, no change in plasma AM levels was seen during a hypertensive attack, although both epinephrine and norepinephrine levels were markedly increased.[23] Subsequent studies also supported the notion that plasma AM levels in the adrenal vein are not increased,[24] which makes it unlikely that the adrenal medulla is a significant source of circulating AM. Thus, although expression of AM peptide and mRNA is widely distributed in various tissues and organs, the main source of plasma AM is now thought to be the vasculature, as AM mRNA is more prominently expressed in vascular endothelial cells and smooth muscle cells than in the adrenal gland.[25,26]

The plasma half-life of AM is reportedly 22.0 ± 1.6 min, with a metabolic clearance rate of 27.4 ± 3.6 mL/kg per minute and with an apparent volume of distribution of 880 ± 150 mL/kg.[27] It appears likely that AM is initially degraded by metalloproteases to yield AM [8–52], AM [26–52] and AM [33–52], followed by aminopeptidase action yielding AM [2–52], AM [27–52], and AM [28–52].[28] The lung appears to be a major site of AM clearance in humans.[23] We also reported that active AM-mature is specifically extracted from the pulmonary circulation.[19,29] Neutral endopeptidase is localized in greatest abundance in the kidney, where it cleaves endogenous peptides that, like AM, possesses a disulfide ring. Lisy and colleagues[30] reported that inhibition of neutral endopeptidase potentiates the natriuretic actions of exogenous AM in anesthetized dogs, suggesting that AM is also degraded by neutral endopeptidase.

Plasma Adrenomedullin Levels in Heart Failure

Several reports have shown that plasma AM levels increase in heart failure in proportion the disease severity.[31–33] We also previously reported on plasma AM levels in heart failure and on the relationships between the levels of AM and other neurohumoral factors in plasma, including atrial natriuretic peptide (ANP), brain (or B-type) natriuretic peptide (BNP), and norepinephrine.[31] We detected no increase of plasma AM levels in patients with New York Heart Association (NYHA) class I, but levels were slightly but significantly increased in patients with NYHA class II, and they were further increased in NYHA class III or IV (**Fig. 2**).[31] Plasma AM levels correlated positively with the ANP and BNP levels and correlated negatively with the left ventricular ejection fraction. After administering treatment for heart failure, plasma ANP and BNP rapidly decreased, but AM levels decreased more slowly.[31] These results indicate that plasma AM levels increase in proportion to disease severity and that they change more slowly than ANP or

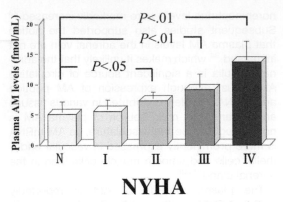

Fig. 2. Plasma AM levels in patients with heart failure in NYHA functional classes I, II, III, and IV and in healthy subjects (N).

BNP levels, which is consistent with other recent reports.[34]

Hirayama and colleagues[35] reported that both AM-mature and AM-glycine, the inactive and major circulating AM form,[14,17] are similarly increased in patients with heart failure. This suggests AM responds to the pathophysiology of heart failure and may be a biomarker indicative of heart failure severity. Subsequent reports support this hypothesis and show that the plasma AM level is an independent prognostic indicator of mild to moderate heart failure[36] and of ischemic heart failure with established ischemic left ventricular dysfunction.[37] Thus, in addition to being an important biomarker for evaluating the severity of heart failure, AM may also be a prognostic indicator for this ailment.

Plasma Mid-Regional Pro-Adrenomedullin Levels as a Prognostic Indicator of Heart Failure

Using a recently developed MR-proAM assay,[12] Gegenhuber and colleagues[38] compared the utility of BNP and MR-proAM as prognostic markers in 137 patients with acute decompensated heart failure. Receiver operating characteristic (ROC) curve analysis showed that the areas under curve for prediction of 1-year mortality were similar for BNP and MR-proAM. In addition, Kaplan-Meier curve analyses showed that the predictive values of BNP and MR-proAM with respect to survival were comparable, and multivariable Cox proportional-hazards regression analyses revealed that increases in the BNP and MR-proAM concentrations were the 2 strongest predictors of mortality. Thus, the predictive properties of MR-proAM measurements appear to be similar to those of BNP in acute decompensated heart failure.

von Haehling and colleagues[39] assessed MR-proAM in 501 patients with chronic heart failure and showed that it increased with NYHA class. Moreover, increases in MR-proAM were predictive of poor survival at 12 months. ROC curve analysis showed that the areas under the curve for MR-proAM and NT-proBNP were similar, whereas Cox proportional hazard analysis showed that both NT-proBNP and MR-proAM added prognostic value to a base model using left ventricular ejection fraction, age, creatinine, and NYHA class. Adding MR-proAM to the base model gave stronger prognostic power than adding NT-proBNP. Thus, MR-proAM is an independent predictor of mortality in patients with chronic heart failure, which adds prognostic information to NT-proBNP.

Maisel and colleagues[40] assessed the prognostic value of MR-proAM in a 15-center, international study of 1641 patients presenting to the emergency department with dyspnea (Biomarkers in Acute Heart Failure [BACH] trial). Using cutoff values from ROC analyses, the accuracy of 90-day survival predictions for patients with heart failure was 73% for MR-proAM and 62% for BNP, which suggests MR-proAM is a more accurate predictor of 90-day mortality than BNP. In an adjusted multivariable Cox regression, MR-proAM, but not BNP, carried independent prognostic value. Thus, MR-proAM identifies patients at high 90-day mortality risk and adds prognostic value to BNP. Using the BACH trial dataset, Maisel and colleagues[41] also evaluated the prognostic accuracy of MR-proAM for 90-day mortality in all enrolled patients. They found that MR-proAM was superior to BNP or troponin for predicting 90-day all-cause mortality in patients presenting with acute dyspnea. Furthermore, MR-proAM added significantly to all clinical variables and was superior to all other biomarkers. In addition, serial evaluation of MR-proAM in patients admitted provided significant added value over a model using admission values only. Finally, those investigators also showed that patients initially at high risk could be identified as low-risk patients through biomarker evaluation at discharge. This suggests MR-proAM may be useful for identifying patients at high 90-day mortality risk and for adding prognostic value to BNP in patients with dyspnea. Serial measurement of MR-proAM may also prove useful for monitoring patients' condition.[41]

Another acute heart failure study by Shah and colleagues[42] assessed the diagnostic and prognostic value of mid-regional pro-ANP (MR-proANP) and MR-proAM in 560 patients presenting with acute dyspnea. Plasma MR-proANP levels were higher in patients with acute decompensated heart failure and remained an independent predictor of heart failure diagnosis. In time-dependent analyses, MR-proAM had the highest area under the curve for death during the first year. Both MR-proAM and MR-proANP were independently prognostic and reclassified risk at 1 year and at 4 years, and in Kaplan-Meier curves both mid-regional peptides were associated with death out to 4 years. Thus, MR-proANP is accurate for diagnosis of acute decompensated heart failure, while both MR-proAM and MR-proANP are independently prognostic over 4 years of follow-up.

To investigate whether MR-proAM is predictive of long-term all-cause mortality in stable outpatients, 724 such stable outpatients were followed for 6 years, during which there were 195 deaths. MR-proAM was predictive of mortality in the overall patient population, and its predictive value for long-term mortality was independent of BNP and other indices. These results suggest that MR-proAM is a potent independent predictor of long-term all-cause mortality in both patients with acute heart failure and stable outpatients.[43]

A recent study investigated whether MR-proAM could provide diagnostic and prognostic information for 311 patients with acute dyspnea. MR-proAM levels at the time of hospital admission were higher in patients with acute heart failure than patients hospitalized with non–heart failure–related dyspnea. The ROC area under the curve for MR-proADM to diagnose heart failure was 0.77 and 0.86 for NT-proBNP. During a median follow-up of 816 days, 66 of 143 patients with acute heart failure and 35 of 84 patients with acute exacerbation of chronic obstructive pulmonary disease (AECOPD) died. In multivariate Cox regression analyses, MR-proAM levels at the time of admission were associated with mortality in patients with acute heart failure, but not in those with AECOPD. MR-proAM levels on admission also improved risk stratification in acute heart failure, as assessed from the net reclassification index. Thus, whereas MR-proAM levels at the time of admission provide strong prognostic information about patients with acute heart failure, they provide only modest diagnostic information for patients with acute dyspnea, which is consistent with previous reports.[44]

The results summarized previously suggest that higher MR-proAM levels are associated with greater risk of mortality and morbidity in patients with acute and chronic heart failure. Indeed, MR-proAM may outperform all other established markers for identification of patients at highest risk of death. It may therefore be useful to include AM and/or MR-proAM measurements in the routine clinical workup of patients with heart failure.

Pathophysiological Significance of Plasma Adrenomedullin in Heart Failure

As mentioned, plasma AM levels increase in proportion to the severity of heart failure and correlate modestly with plasma ANP and BNP levels. However, the diagnostic accuracy of AM for heart failure is modest. After treatment, plasma AM levels decline only slowly on improvement of the heart failure condition. On the other hand, the significance of AM as a prognostic marker in heart failure is strong and reportedly stronger than BNP. Plasma AM originates from multiple organs and tissues, particularly blood vessels. So why is AM more strongly related to prognosis in heart failure than BNP? This may reflect that the cause of death in heart failure is not related solely to the heart. Inflammation is deeply involved in the pathophysiology of heart failure.[45] Heart failure progresses, at least in part, as a result of the deleterious effects of endogenous cytokine cascades on the heart and peripheral circulation. In various tissues, AM mRNA is strongly induced by cytokines,[25,26,46] suggesting plasma AM concentrations may reflect cytokine upregulation in peripheral tissues. In addition, the cause of death in heart failure is often related to infectious diseases such as pneumonia and septicemia,[47] and the AM gene is also strongly induced by such infections.[48] Of course, cardiac AM expression is also increased in heart failure.[49] Thus, given that plasma AM reflects the systemic pathologic condition in heart failure, plasma AM may be superior to plasma BNP as a prognostic predictor.

SUMMARY

AM is closely related to the pathophysiology of heart failure. Because increased plasma AM levels are predictive of a poor prognosis, it can be a useful biomarker for detecting heart failure patients at high risk.

ACKNOWLEDGMENTS

The authors thank Yukari Kubo for her excellent secretarial work.

REFERENCES

1. Schrier RW, Abraham WT. Hormones and hemodynamics in heart failure. N Engl J Med 1999;341: 577–85.
2. Kitamura K, Kangawa K, Kawamoto M, et al. Adrenomedullin: a novel hypotensive peptide isolated

from human pheochromocytoma. Biochem Biophys Res Commun 1993;192:553–60.

3. Kitamura K, Sakata J, Kangawa K, et al. Cloning and characterization of cDNA encoding a precursor for human adrenomedullin. Biochem Biophys Res Commun 1993;194:720–5.

4. Nishikimi T, Matsuoka H. Cardiac adrenomedullin: its role in cardiac hypertrophy and heart failure. Curr Med Chem Cardiovasc Hematol Agents 2005;3: 231–42.

5. Nishikimi T. Adrenomedullin in the kidney-renal physiological and pathophysiological roles. Curr Med Chem 2007;14:1689–99.

6. Nishikimi T, Kuwahara K, Nakagawa Y, et al. Adrenomedullin in cardiovascular disease: a useful biomarker, its pathological roles and therapeutic application. Curr Protein Pept Sci 2013;14:256–67.

7. Nagaya N, Nishikimi T, Horio T, et al. Cardiovascular and renal effects of adrenomedullin in rats with heart failure. Am J Physiol 1999;276:R213–8.

8. Nishikimi T, Karasawa T, Inaba C, et al. Effects of long-term intravenous administration of adrenomedullin (AM) plus hANP therapy in acute decompensated heart failure: a pilot study. Circ J 2009;73: 892–8.

9. Kitamura K, Ichiki Y, Tanaka M, et al. Immunoreactive adrenomedullin in human plasma. FEBS Lett 1994;341:288–90.

10. Kohno M, Hanehira T, Kano H, et al. Plasma adrenomedullin concentrations in essential hypertension. Hypertension 1996;27:102–7.

11. Lewis LK, Smith MW, Yandle TG, et al. Adrenomedullin(1-52) measured in human plasma by radioimmunoassay: plasma concentration, adsorption, and storage. Clin Chem 1998;44:571–7.

12. Christ-Crain M, Morgenthaler NG, Struck J, et al. Mid-regional pro-adrenomedullin as a prognostic marker in sepsis: an observational study. Crit Care 2005;9:R816–24.

13. Nishikimi T, Horio T, Kohmoto Y, et al. Molecular forms of plasma and urinary adrenomedullin in normal, essential hypertension and chronic renal failure. J Hypertens 2001;19:765–73.

14. Kitamura K, Kato J, Kawamoto M, et al. The intermediate form of glycine-extended adrenomedullin is the major circulating molecular form in human plasma. Biochem Biophys Res Commun 1998;244: 551–5.

15. Ohta H, Tsuji T, Asai S, et al. One-step direct assay for mature-type adrenomedullin with monoclonal antibodies. Clin Chem 1999;45:244–51.

16. Ohta H, Tsuji T, Asai S, et al. A simple immunoradiometric assay for measuring the entire molecules of adrenomedullin in human plasma. Clin Chim Acta 1999;287:131–43.

17. Nishikimi T, Matsuoka H, Shimada K, et al. Production and clearance sites of two molecular forms of adrenomedullin in human plasma. Am J Hypertens 2000;13:1032–4.

18. Asakawa H, Nishikimi T, Suzuki T, et al. Elevation of two molecular forms of adrenomedullin in plasma and urine in patients with acute myocardial infarction treated with early coronary angioplasty. Clin Sci 2001;100:117–26.

19. Nishikimi T, Nagata S, Sasaki T, et al. The active molecular form of plasma adrenomedullin is extracted in the pulmonary circulation in patients with mitral stenosis: possible role of adrenomedullin in pulmonary hypertension. Clin Sci (Lond) 2001;100:61–6.

20. Tadokoro K, Nishikimi T, Mori Y, et al. Altered gene expression of adrenomedullin and its receptor system and molecular forms of tissue adrenomedullin in left ventricular hypertrophy induced by malignant hypertension. Regul Pept 2003;112:71–8.

21. Nishikimi T, Tadokoro K, Mori Y, et al. Ventricular adrenomedullin system in the transition from LVH to heart failure in rats. Hypertension 2003;41:512–8.

22. Wang X, Nishikimi T, Akimoto K, et al. Upregulation of ligand, receptor system, and amidating activity of adrenomedullin in left ventricular hypertrophy of severely hypertensive rats: effects of angiotensin-converting enzyme inhibitors and diuretic. J Hypertens 2003;21:1171–81.

23. Nishikimi T, Kitamura K, Saito Y, et al. Clinical studies on the sites of production and clearance of circulating adrenomedullin in human subjects. Hypertension 1994;24:600–4.

24. Minami J, Nishikimi T, Todoroki M, et al. Source of plasma adrenomedullin in patients with pheochromocytoma. Am J Hypertens 2002;15:994–7.

25. Sugo S, Minamino N, Kangawa K, et al. Endothelial cells actively synthesize and secrete adrenomedullin. Biochem Biophys Res Commun 1994;201: 1160–6.

26. Sugo S, Minamino N, Shoji H, et al. Production and secretion of adrenomedullin from vascular smooth muscle cells: augmented production by tumor necrosis factor-alpha. Biochem Biophys Res Commun 1994;203:719–26.

27. Meeran K, O'Shea D, Upton PD, et al. Circulating adrenomedullin does not regulate systemic blood pressure but increases plasma prolactin after intravenous infusion in humans: a pharmacokinetic study. J Clin Endocrinol Metab 1997;82:95–100.

28. Lewis LK, Smith MW, Brennan SO, et al. Degradation of human adrenomedullin(1-52) by plasma membrane enzymes and identification of metabolites. Peptides 1997;18:733–9.

29. Watanabe K, Nishikimi T, Takamuro M, et al. Two molecular forms of adrenomedullin in congenital heart disease. Pediatr Cardiol 2003;24:559–65.

30. Lisy O, Jougasaki M, Schirger JA, et al. Neutral endopeptidase inhibition potentiates the natriuretic

actions of adrenomedullin. Am J Physiol 1998;275: F410–4.

31. Nishikimi T, Saito Y, Kitamura K, et al. Increased plasma levels of adrenomedullin in patients with heart failure. J Am Coll Cardiol 1995;26:1424–31.

32. Jougasaki M, Wei CM, McKinley LJ, et al. Elevation of circulating and ventricular adrenomedullin in human congestive heart failure. Circulation 1995;92: 286–9.

33. Kato J, Kobayashi K, Etoh T, et al. Plasma adrenomedullim concentration in patients with heart failure. J Clin Endocrinol Metab 1996;81:180–3.

34. Boyer B, Hart KW, Sperling MI, et al. Biomarker changes during acute heart failure treatment. Congest Heart Fail 2012;18:91–7.

35. Hirayama N, Kitamura K, Imamura T, et al. Molecular forms of circulating adrenomedullin in patients with congestive heart failure. J Endocrinol 1999;160: 297–303.

36. Pousset F, Masson F, Chavirovskaia O, et al. Plasma adrenomedullin, a new independent predictor of prognosis in patients with chronic heart failure. Eur Heart J 2000;21:1009–14.

37. Richards AM, Doughty R, Nicholls MG, et al, Australia-New Zealand Heart Failure Group. Plasma N-terminal pro-brain natriuretic peptide and adrenomedullin: prognostic utility and prediction of benefit from carvedilol in chronic ischemic left ventricular dysfunction. Australia-New Zealand Heart Failure Group. J Am Coll Cardiol 2001;37:1781–7.

38. Gegenhuber A, Struck J, Dieplinger B, et al. Comparative evaluation of B-type natriuretic peptide, mid-regional pro-A-type natriuretic peptide, mid-regional pro-adrenomedullin, and Copeptin to predict 1-year mortality in patients with acute destabilized heart failure. J Card Fail 2007;13:42–9.

39. von Haehling S, Filippatos GS, Papassotiriou J, et al. Mid-regional pro-adrenomedullin as a novel predictor of mortality in patients with chronic heart failure. Eur J Heart Fail 2010;12:484–91.

40. Maisel A, Mueller C, Nowak R, et al. Mid-region prohormone markers for diagnosis and prognosis in acute dyspnea: results from the BACH (Biomarkers in Acute Heart Failure) trial. J Am Coll Cardiol 2010;1:2062–76.

41. Maisel A, Mueller C, Nowak RM, et al. Midregion prohormone adrenomedullin and prognosis in patients presenting with acute dyspnea: results from the BACH (Biomarkers in Acute Heart Failure) trial. J Am Coll Cardiol 2011;58:1057–67.

42. Shah RV, Truong QA, Gaggin HK, et al. Mid-regional pro-atrial natriuretic peptide and pro-adrenomedullin testing for the diagnostic and prognostic evaluation of patients with acute dyspnoea. Eur Heart J 2012;33:2197–205.

43. Xue Y, Taub P, Iqbal N, et al. Mid-region pro-adrenomedullin adds predictive value to clinical predictors and Framingham risk score for long-term mortality in stable outpatients with heart failure. Eur J Heart Fail 2013;15:1343–9.

44. Pervez MO, Lyngbakken MN, Myhre PL, et al. Mid-regional pro-adrenomedullin in patients with acute dyspnea: data from the Akershus Cardiac Examination (ACE) 2 Study. Clin Biochem 2017;50: 394–400.

45. Mann DL. Innate immunity and the failing heart: cytokine hypothesis revisited. Circ Res 2015;116: 1254–68.

46. Horio T, Nishikimi T, Yoshihara F, et al. Production and secretion of adrenomedullin in cultured rat cardiac myocytes and nonmyocytes: stimulation by interleukin-1beta and tumor necrosis factor-alpha. Endocrinology 1998;139:4576–80.

47. Lee DS, Gona P, Albano I, et al. A systematic assessment of causes of death after heart failure onset in the community: impact of age at death, time period, and left ventricular systolic dysfunction. Circ Heart Fail 2011;4:36–43.

48. Nishio K, Akai Y, Murao Y, et al. Increased plasma concentrations of adrenomedullin correlate with relaxation of vascular tone in patients with septic shock. Crit Care Med 1997;25:953–7.

49. Nishikimi T, Horio T, Sasaki T, et al. Cardiac production and secretion of adrenomedullin are increased in heart failure. Hypertension 1997;30:1369–75.

Troponin in Heart Failure

Kevin S. Shah, MD[a,*], Alan S. Maisel, MD[b], Gregg C. Fonarow, MD[c]

KEYWORDS

- Troponin • Heart failure • Prognosis • Biomarker • Mortality

KEY POINTS

- Troponin is often elevated in patients with chronic and acute heart failure, with and without coexisting coronary artery disease.
- As high sensitive assays become more common in clinical practice, more patients with heart failure will have detectable troponin.
- Measuring high sensitive troponin in patients at risk for heart disease does provide additional predictive ability regarding incident heart failure.
- Troponin elevation in acute, chronic heart failure with reduced and preserved ejection fraction has prognostic value for future poor outcomes.

INTRODUCTION

Measurement and interpretation of cardiac troponin (cTn) is an integral part of the management of patients with acute coronary syndrome (ACS).[1] A rise-and-fall pattern of cTn is a part of the diagnostic criteria for acute myocardial infarction (AMI), and elevated cTn provides prognostic value in multiple noncardiac conditions.[2] Heart failure (HF) is a chronic, progressive condition that affects an estimated 5.7 million Americans.[3] It is a rising global epidemic with greater than 37.7 million affected worldwide.[4,5] Older individuals are particularly affected, with over half of patients hospitalized greater than 75 years of age.[6] Biomarkers play an critical role in the management of patients with or at risk for HF.[7] The American Heart Association (AHA) recently published a scientific statement regarding the role of biomarkers in the management of HF.[7] The role of troponin in the management of patients with HF is evolving with a growing body of evidence for its potential. In this review, the authors discuss the role of troponin in prediction, management, and prognostication of patients with HF. Specifically, the authors detail the unique role in acute and chronic HF, as well differences in reduced ejection fraction versus preserved ejection fraction HF. Finally, the authors discuss novel data using high sensitive troponin assays and potential strategies in the future to improve the use of troponin in caring for patients with HF.

HEART FAILURE

HF is defined by the American College of Cardiology and the AHA as a complex clinical syndrome that results from any structural or functional impairment of ventricular filling or ejection of blood.[8] The result is a constellation of signs and symptoms related to either congestion or low cardiac output. HF is most often subtyped in to 2 categories: reduced or preserved ejection fraction (HFrEF or HFpEF, respectively).

Disclosure Statement: Dr K.S. Shah has no relevant conflicts of interest to disclose. Dr A.S. Maisel reported serving as a consultant to Critical Diagnostics and Alere. Dr G.C. Fonarow reported serving as a consultant to Janssen Pharmaceutical and Novartis.
a University of California, Los Angeles, 650 Charles E. Young Drive South, A2-237 CHS, MC: 167917, Los Angeles, CA 90095, USA; b Division of Cardiology, UC San Diego, 3350 La Jolla Village Drive, San Diego, CA 92161, USA; c Division of Cardiology, Department of Medicine, Ronald Reagan UCLA Medical Center, 10833 LeConte Avenue, Room A2-237 CHS, Los Angeles, CA 90095-1679, USA
* Corresponding author.
E-mail address: kshah@mednet.ucla.edu

Heart Failure Clin 14 (2018) 57–64
http://dx.doi.org/10.1016/j.hfc.2017.08.007
1551-7136/18/© 2017 Elsevier Inc. All rights reserved.

The cause of HF can vary, with higher income regions frequently affected by ischemic heart disease and low-income regions by hypertensive, rheumatic and myocarditis.[5] An analysis of 24 large HF trials demonstrated coronary artery disease (CAD) was the underlying cause in nearly 65% of patients.[9] The importance and relevance of cTn in HF not only lies in those with ischemic HF but also non-ischemic HF. The burden of HF is large, with the direct costs and prevalence of HF estimated to increase by 200% and 25%, respectively, over the next 20 years.[10,11] Thus, there exists a need for additional tools to help improve care for this costly and high-risk population.

TROPONIN

Troponin proteins are involved in the regulation of cardiac muscle contraction. Troponin I (inhibitory), troponin C (calcium binding) and troponin T (tropomyosin binding) proteins form the troponin complex.[12] There are variable isoforms of each subtype of troponin found within cardiac and skeletal muscle. Although most cTn is part of the contractile apparatus, some troponin I (cTnI) and troponin T (cTnT) is found free in the cytosol.[13] Detectable levels of cTnI and cTnT in the serum are always found in patients with myocardial infarction with a typical rise-and-fall pattern. This elevation in cTn is part of the diagnostic criteria for acute myocardial infarction.[14] Clinical assays exist for the detection of cTnT and cTnI with varying degrees of sensitivity and limits of detection. More recently, high sensitive assays have been developed and routinely used in clinical practice; these detect cTn levels to nanogram and picogram levels. To be considered a high sensitive assay, detectable cTn should be found in greater than 50% of healthy subjects.[2,15] A high sensitive troponin assay (Roche) was recently approved by the Food and Drug Administration for use in the United States. Most studies of the utility of cTn in HF were performed with contemporary sensitive assays, although the volume of data regarding high sensitive cTn (hs-cTn) is growing.

MECHANISMS OF CARDIAC TROPONIN ELEVATION IN HEART FAILURE

There are multiple theories as to why patients with HF have detectable cTn. The most prevailing theory is related to persistent subendocardial ischemia, which may or may not be related to epicardial obstructive CAD.[16] In acute decompensated HF, reduced cardiac output and increased ventricular filling pressures can worsen the coronary perfusion gradient. These mechanisms lead to cardiac ischemia and release of cTn. In chronic HF, continuous upregulation of the renin-angiotensin aldosterone system may lead to persistent cell injury and death. Detectable cTn has been consistently found in patients with ischemic and nonischemic HF.[17] In patients with nonischemic HF, there is an association with cTn and a restrictive mitral Doppler pattern as well as left ventricular (LV) concentric remodeling.[16] When cTn is elevated in a new case of acute HF (AHF), it is often questioned as to whether ischemia was the trigger for the episode itself or if cTn release is sequelae from the decompensated state. Serial measurements and clinical history are imperative in distinguishing between these two hypotheses. Other theories as to the mechanism behind cTn release in HF include myocyte damage from inflammatory cytokines or oxidative stress,[18] apoptosis of hibernating myocardium,[19] or injured myocardium and permeable membranes with leakage.[20] As the sensitivity for cTn assays have improved, many acute conditions, including sepsis, arrhythmia, hypertension, cardiotoxicity from chemotherapy, and renal failure, have associated elevated cTn.[21]

TROPONIN TO PREDICT INCIDENT HEART FAILURE

In patients without a diagnosis of HF, multiple biomarkers have shown an association with the development of future HF. Biomarkers, such as soluble ST-2, growth differentiation factor 15, and natriuretic peptides, have shown modest predictive ability in the Framingham Heart Study to predict incident HF.[22–24] Troponin as a marker of underlying myocyte dysfunction may also have potential as a predictor of new HF. Chronic and low-level myocyte injury may be ongoing in individuals, which can precede the development of clinical HF. DeFilippi and colleagues[25] studied the role of hs-cTnT in 4221 subjects older than 65 years from the Cardiovascular Heart Study cohort. From the cohort, 66.2% of subjects had baseline detectable cTnT. The baseline and an increase from the baseline to 2 years' follow-up both were associated with the development of HF. When added to a prediction model (including demographics, clinical risk factors, medications, and biomarkers N-terminal pro b-type natriuretic peptide and C-reactive protein), hs-cTnT provided a modest addition to a risk prediction for future HF. A similar analysis by Saunders and colleagues[26] studying the Atherosclerosis Risk in Community (ARIC) cohort demonstrated measurable cTnT in

66.5% of subjects; elevated cTnT was associated with eventual hospitalization for HF. Based on these data, there is evidence that measurement of cTn and monitoring of long-term serial changes in a general population can help identify individuals at risk for HF.

TROPONIN AS A PREDICTOR OF NEW HEART FAILURE AFTER MYOCARDIAL INFARCTION

A new diagnosis of HF in the setting of AMI is a frequent occurrence, with some studies citing evidence of new LV dysfunction at 40%.[27] Often, new HF is detected in the evaluation of ACS; management of both conditions occur in parallel. In the setting of AMI, ventricular remodeling occurs at variable degrees depending on infarct size/location. In one analysis, among patients with AMI, 62.7% developed HF in the 6 years following their initial event.[28] Peak cTnT correlates well with infarct size in patients with AMI.[29] The Long-Term Intervention with Pravastatin in Ischemic Disease (LIPID) study followed patients after an ACS event for the development of adverse events. Patients who had an increase from baseline to 1 year of cTn (measured by a contemporary assay) had an association with HF hospitalization.[30] Similarly, Gerber and colleagues[31] demonstrated that cTnT elevation was associated with development of HF 2 years after an AMI, with a dose-response pattern (higher levels having greater association with HF). In summary, patients who experience AMI are at increased risk for future development of HF. There is a relationship between degree of cTn elevation, infarct size, and long-term progression to clinical HF. Attention should be paid to patients with elevated cTn in this setting to identify patients who may benefit from closer surveillance for the development of either clinical HF or asymptomatic LV dysfunction.

TROPONIN AND ACUTE HEART FAILURE

Most literature regarding cTn in HF has been published on the value of detectable cTn in the AHF setting. Peacock and colleagues[32] examined the prognostic value of baseline cTn in patients with AHF in a landmark article from the Acute Decompensated Heart Failure National Registry (ADHERE). Of 67,924 patients, 4240 patients (6.2%) had elevated cTnT or cTnI on admission for AHF. Troponin-positive patients had a higher rate of in-hospital mortality than troponin-negative patients (8.0% vs 2.7%, $P<.001$). In addition, the patients with elevated baseline cTn had more frequent adverse inpatient events and increased in-hospital mortality, independently of

treatment. Finally, in this analysis, troponin-positive patients were more likely to be receiving nitroglycerin, inotropic agents, and vasodilator therapy. These findings likely represent a more ill patient population, as patients with elevated cTn also required more time in the intensive care unit (ICU).

In the Acute Study of Clinical Effectiveness of Nesiritide in Decompensated Heart Failure (ASCEND-HF) trial, 78% of patients had detectable cTn and 50% of patients had cTnI greater than the 99th percentile.[33] Patients with ischemic and nonischemic HF had no difference in cTn; however, patients with HFrEF had greater cTn than HFpEF. These elevations were also associated with worsened in-hospital length of stay, worsened HF, and death but did not have prognostic value after discharge from the hospital. Interestingly, subjects who had serial inpatient measurement of cTn with an increase or falling pattern more than or less than the 99th percentile did not have a difference in their short-term mortality. This large analysis (n = 808) reemphasized the prognostic implications of cTn during inpatient hospitalization for HF but differed with other studies given no long-term association with adverse outcomes.

With respect to high sensitive troponin, analyses specifically using novel assays for AHF have been performed. Given the fact that hs-cTn assays are associated with more individuals with detectable cTn in healthy individuals, there are likely more patients with HF with elevated hs-cTn. Parissis and colleagues[34] performed a small analysis of patients with undetectable contemporary cTn but positive hs-cTn with AHF. Patients had follow-up after hospitalization for a median period of 174 days. A cutoff of hs-cTn greater than 77 pg/mL identified patients with a worse long-term prognosis. Additionally, in an undifferentiated cohort of dyspneic patients in the emergency department, subjects diagnosed with AHF with elevated hs-cTn from the Basics in Acute Shortness of Breath Evaluation (BASEL) study had an increased risk of short- and long-term mortality.[35] Arenja and colleagues[35] demonstrated that patients with AHF with increasing cTn had a higher likelihood of ICU admission, in-hospital death, and short-term death. Xue and colleagues[36] studied patients undergoing treatment of AHF; those who had increasing hs-cTn despite HF therapy also had increased mortality. These studies demonstrate that elevated cTn measured at baseline and serially in patients with AHF is independently associated with short-term outcomes. Furthermore, the use of high sensitive assays detects cTn in patients with AHF who are also at increased risk but have normal cTn by a contemporary assay. In patients whose cTn increases during acute treatment of HF, they are at high risk for adverse long-term outcomes.

TROPONIN AND CHRONIC HEART FAILURE

Multiple large trials of patients with chronic HF have studied the prognostic value of cTn. In the Valsartan Heart Failure Trial (Val-HeFT) trial, baseline cTn was measured in 4053 patients.[37] Baseline cTn was elevated in 10.4% of patients, and cTn correlated with the New York Heart Association (NYHA) stage of HF. Furthermore, cTn was associated with long-term mortality after 2 years. In addition, the investigators measured hs-cTn, which was detectable in 92.0% of patients. Elevated hs-cTn was associated with long-term mortality and HF hospitalization. In a multivariate model, hs-cTn added to the ability of clinical variables and brain natriuretic peptide (BNP) to predict long-term mortality. Grodin and colleagues[38] also analyzed cTn and hs-cTn in patients with chronic HF. In patients with elevated cTn and hs-cTn, higher hs-cTn was associated with a 2-fold increase in 5-year mortality after adjusting for traditional HF risk factors (**Fig. 1**). Jungbauer and colleagues[39] also found that elevated hs-cTn in patients with chronic HFrEF was associated with long-term mortality as well as rehospitalization for HF.[39] Gravning and colleagues[40] studied the value of hs-cTn in elderly (>60 years) patients with chronic ischemic HF. Similarly, hs-cTn had a strong predictive all-cause and cardiovascular (CV) mortality. In their analysis, the baseline value was superior to changes of hs-cTn during follow-up. Nagarajan and colleagues[41] performed a meta-analysis of studies analyzing cTn in chronic HF and concluded there was no significant difference between high and low sensitivity cTn in terms of long-term outcomes. To summarize, multiple large studies have demonstrated a strong association with cTn (regardless of assay) for mortality and adverse short- and long-term outcomes in patients with chronic HF. **Table 1** summarizes recent studies using cTn to assess prognosis in patients with HF.

TROPONIN AND HEART FAILURE WITH PRESERVED EJECTION FRACTION

Pandey and colleagues[42] performed an analysis from the Get With The Guidelines (GWTG) registry to evaluate the prognostic ability of hs-cTn (cTnI and cTnT) in patients with HFpEF. Prior studies had demonstrated cTn is generally lower in HFpEF than in HFrEF.[43] From the GWTG analysis of 34,233 patients, clinical factors associated with an cTn included older age, black race, elevated creatinine, elevated BNP, smoking, ischemic heart disease, elevated heart rate, and systolic blood pressure. Furthermore, those with elevated hs-cTn had higher rates of in-hospital mortality and length of stay. Long-term, these patients also had a higher incidence of 30-day death/readmission and 1-year death. The investigators concluded more routine use of cTn measurement in patients with decompensated HFpEF may identify the highest-risk patients. It further underscores the recurring finding in studies that elevated hs-cTn is a poor prognostic marker in many clinical scenarios, including decompensated HFpEF.

TROPONIN AND ADVANCED HEART FAILURE AND TRANSPLANT CARDIOLOGY

In patients who have undergone cardiac transplant, the process of monitoring for chronic graft rejection is multifaceted, including imaging, endomyocardial biopsy, and blood testing. Dengler and

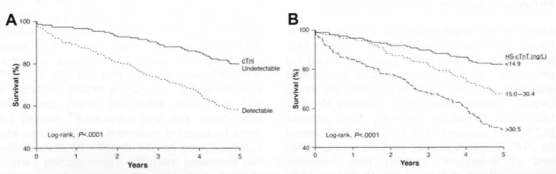

Fig. 1. (*A*) Kaplan-Meier estimates of 5-year survival rates according to cTnI levels more than or less than the limit of detection. (*B*) Kaplan-Meier estimates of 5-year survival rates according to hs-cTnT levels. (*From* Grodin JL, Neale S, Wu Y, et al. Prognostic comparison of different sensitivity cardiac troponin assays in stable heart failure. Am J Med 2015;128:276–82; with permission.)

Table 1
Recent studies analyzing prognosis in patients with heart failure and elevated cardiac troponin

Author, Reference, Year	N	Troponin	HF Type	Outcome	Multivariate Adjusted
Peacock et al,[32] 2008	67,924	Contemporary cTnT and cTnI	AHF	In-hospital mortality	Yes
Felker et al,[33] 2012	808	Contemporary cTnI	AHF	In-hospital length of stay or worsening HF	Yes
Parissis et al,[34] 2013	113	hs-cTnT	AHF	Long-term mortality	Yes
Arenja et al,[35] 2012	667	hs-cTnI	AHF	Short- and long-term mortality	Yes
Xue et al,[36] 2011	144	hs-cTnI	AHF	Short-term HF rehospitalization and mortality	Yes
Latini et al,[37] 2007	4053	hs-cTnT	CHF	Long-term mortality and HF hospitalization	Yes
Grodin et al,[38] 2015	504	hs-cTnT and contemporary cTnI	CHF	Long-term mortality	Yes
Jungbauer et al,[39] 2011	233	hs-cTnT	CHF	Long-term mortality and rehospitalization	Yes
Gravning et al,[40] 2014	1245	hs-cTnT	Chronic ischemic HF	CV death, nonfatal myocardial infarction, and nonfatal stroke	Yes
Pandey et al,[42] 2016	34,233	Contemporary cTnT and cTnI	AHF (HFpEF)	In-hospital mortality, greater length of stay, 30-d and 1-y mortality	Yes

colleagues[44] demonstrated that in acute allograft rejection, cTnT is elevated and correlates with severity of graft rejection. In a small study of 100 patients who had undergone a heart transplant, 37 patients had detectable cTnT with a high-sensitive assay. These patients had a greater incidence of transplant coronary vasculopathy as well as posttransplant HF.[45] Another study of 108 transplant patients demonstrated a combination of hs-cTnT and mean myocardial perfusion reserve predicted death and need for revascularization.[46] Although it is a smaller patient population, cTn has shown some value in the posttransplant setting, particularly as an additional tool in monitoring for complications. To date, there has been little research performed on patients with advanced HF who have undergone implantation of mechanical circulatory support devices and cTn.

FUTURE DIRECTIONS

The most important addition a biomarker can provide in clinical care is the ability to affect management and ultimately clinical outcomes. The ideal biomarker is either sensitive or specific and may have an effect on decision-making. As high sensitive assays become more abundant in routine practice, more patients with HF will have detectable cTn. The routine measurement of cTn in patients at risk for HF has been shown to have some predictive ability with the development of HF. The next step would be an intervention (ie, tailored lifestyle modification with aggressive risk factor modification) based on identification of these subjects to prevent the development of HF (**Fig. 2**).

In the West of Scotland Coronary Prevention Study (WOSCOPS), Ford and colleagues[47] demonstrated that patients taking pravastatin had a reduction in their measurable hs-cTn and a change at 1 year was associated with coronary risk. This type of potentially actionable data is where the largest clinical benefit would be found with patients with HF. There are multiple therapeutic options between medications and devices for patients with HF, which are often

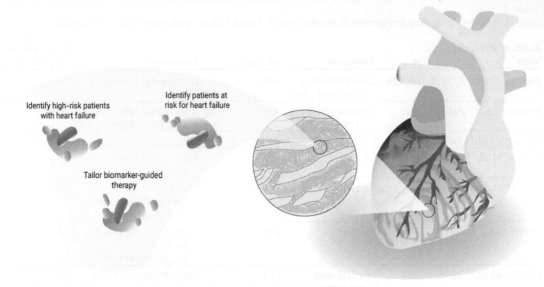

Identify high-risk patients
with heart failure

Identify patients at
risk for heart failure

Tailor biomarker-guided
therapy

Fig. 2. The multiple potential roles of cTn in patients with (or at risk for) HF.

underutilized, between medications and device therapies are considered.[11,48] Individualizing therapies beyond solely ejection fraction and NYHA stage to identify patients is likely where the incremental gains will be had in the future. The use of cTn as an indicator of patients who may respond to certain therapies (ie, anti-ischemic therapy) would be of significant value.

SUMMARY

HF is a deadly and progressive condition. Patients with AHF and chronic HF often have elevated (or positive) troponin. As robust high sensitive troponin assays become more routinely used, more patients with HF will have detectable troponin. Identification of the highest-risk patients using this biomarker among a panel of risk factors will help determine which patients are at risk for future events. Future steps would be to use this biomarker to target individualized therapy to help mitigate the devastating effect of HF.

REFERENCES

1. Roffi M, Patrono C, Collet J-P, et al. 2015 ESC guidelines for the management of acute coronary syndromes in patients presenting without persistent ST-segment elevation. Eur Heart J 2015;32(23): 2999–3054.
2. Xu R-Y, Zhu X-F, Yang Y, et al. High-sensitive cardiac troponin T. J Geriatr Cardiol 2013;10(1):102–9.
3. Mozaffarian D, Benjamin EJ, Go AS, et al. Heart disease and stroke statistics - 2016 update: a report from the American Heart Association. Circulation 2016. http://dx.doi.org/10.1161/CIR.0000000000000350.
4. Bui AL, Horwich TB, Fonarow GC. Epidemiology and risk profile of heart failure. Nat Rev Cardiol 2010; 8(1):30–41.
5. Vos T, Flaxman AD, Naghavi M, et al. Years lived with disability (YLDs) for 1160 sequelae of 289 diseases and injuries 1990-2010: a systematic analysis for the Global Burden of Disease Study 2010. Lancet 2012; 380(9859):2163–96.
6. Chen J, Dharmarajan K, Wang Y, et al. National trends in heart failure hospital stay rates, 2001 to 2009. J Am Coll Cardiol 2013;61(10):1078–88.
7. Chow SL, Maisel AS, Anand I, et al. Role of biomarkers for the prevention, assessment, and management of heart failure: a scientific statement from the American Heart Association. Circulation 2017;135(22):e1054–91.
8. Yancy CW, Jessup M, Bozkurt B, et al. 2013 ACCF/AHA guideline for the management of heart failure: a report of the American College of Cardiology Foundation/American Heart Association Task Force. Circulation 2013;128(16):e240–327. Available at: http://www.ncbi.nlm.nih.gov/pubmed/23741058.
9. Gheorghiade M, Sopko G, De Luca L, et al. Navigating the crossroads of coronary artery disease and heart failure. Circulation 2006;114(11):1202–13.
10. Roger VL. Epidemiology of heart failure. Circ Res 2013;113(6):646–59.
11. Paul S, Lindenfeld J. HFSA 2010 guideline executive summary executive summary: HFSA 2010 comprehensive heart failure practice guideline Heart Failure Society of America. J Card Fail 2010;16:475–539.

12. Parmacek MS, Solaro RJ. Biology of the troponin complex in cardiac myocytes. Prog Cardiovasc Dis 2004;47(3):159–76.

13. Bleier J, Vorderwinkler KP, Falkensammer J, et al. Different intracellular compartmentations of cardiac troponins and myosin heavy chains: a causal connection to their different early release after myocardial damage. Clin Chem 1998;44(9):1912–8.

14. Thygesen K, Alpert JS, Jaffe AS, et al. Third universal definition of myocardial infarction. Eur Heart J 2012;33(20):2551–67.

15. Seydelmann N, Liu D, Krämer J, et al. High-sensitivity troponin: a clinical blood biomarker for staging cardiomyopathy in Fabry disease. J Am Heart Assoc 2016;5(6):e002839.

16. Logeart D, Beyne P, Cusson C, et al. Evidence of cardiac myolysis in severe nonischemic heart failure and the potential role of increased wall strain. Am Heart J 2001;141(2):247–53.

17. Torre M, Jarolim P. Cardiac troponin assays in the management of heart failure. Clin Chim Acta 2014; 441:92–8.

18. Levine B, Kalman J, Mayer L, et al. Elevated circulating levels of tumor necrosis factor in severe chronic heart failure. N Engl J Med 1990;323(4):236–41.

19. Narula J, Haider N, Virmani R, et al. Apoptosis in myocytes in end-stage heart failure. N Engl J Med 1996;335(16):1182–9.

20. Perna ER, Macin SM, Canella JP, et al. Ongoing myocardial injury in stable severe heart failure: value of cardiac troponin T monitoring for high-risk patient identification. Circulation 2004;110(16):2376–82. Available at: http://www.ncbi.nlm.nih.gov/entrez/query.fcgi?cmd=Retrieve&db=PubMed&dopt=Citation&list_uids=15477403.

21. Roongsritong C, Warraich I, Bradley C. Common causes of troponin elevations in the absence of acute myocardial infarction: incidence and clinical significance. Chest 2004;125(5):1877–84.

22. Brouwers FP, Van Gilst WH, Damman K, et al. Clinical risk stratification optimizes value of biomarkers to predict new-onset heart failure in a community-based cohort. Circ Heart Fail 2014;7(5):723–31.

23. Velagaleti RS, Gona P, Larson MG, et al. Multimarker approach for the prediction of heart failure incidence in the community. Circulation 2010; 122(17):1700–6.

24. Parikh RH, Seliger SL, Christenson R, et al. Soluble ST2 for prediction of heart failure and cardiovascular death in an elderly, community-dwelling population. J Am Heart Assoc 2016;5(8):e003188.

25. deFilippi CR, de Lemos JA, Christenson RH, et al. Association of serial measures of cardiac troponin T using a sensitive assay with incident heart failure and cardiovascular mortality in older adults. JAMA 2010;304(22):2494–502.

26. Saunders JT, Nambi V, De Lemos JA, et al. Cardiac troponin T measured by a highly sensitive assay predicts coronary heart disease, heart failure, and mortality in the atherosclerosis risk in communities study. Circulation 2011;123(13):1367–76.

27. Albert NM, Lewis C. Recognizing and managing asymptomatic left ventricular dysfunction: after myocardial infarction. Crit Care Nurse 2008;28(2):20. Available at: http://search.ebscohost.com/login.aspx?direct=true&db=rzh&AN=2009885318&site=ehost-live.

28. Torabi A, Cleland JGF, Khan NK, et al. The timing of development and subsequent clinical course of heart failure after a myocardial infarction. Eur Heart J 2008;29(7):859–70.

29. Hallén J, Buser P, Schwitter J, et al. Relation of cardiac troponin I measurements at 24 and 48 hours to magnetic resonance-determined infarct size in patients with ST-elevation myocardial infarction. Am J Cardiol 2009;104(11):1472–7.

30. White HD, Tonkin A, Simes J, et al. Association of contemporary sensitive troponin i levels at baseline and change at 1 year with long-term coronary events following myocardial infarction or unstable angina: results from the LIPID study (long-term intervention with pravastatin in Ischaemic disease). J Am Coll Cardiol 2014;63(4):345–54.

31. Gerber Y, Jaffe AS, Weston SA, et al. Prognostic value of cardiac troponin T after myocardial infarction: a contemporary community experience. Mayo Clin Proc 2012;87(3):247–54.

32. Peacock WF, De Marco T, Fonarow GC, et al. Cardiac troponin and outcome in acute heart failure. N Engl J Med 2008;358(20):2117–26.

33. Felker GM, Hasselblad V, Tang WH, et al. Troponin i in acute decompensated heart failure: Insights from the ASCEND-HF study. Eur J Heart Fail 2012;14(11):1257–64.

34. Parissis JT, Papadakis J, Kadoglou NPE, et al. Prognostic value of high sensitivity troponin T in patients with acutely decompensated heart failure and non-detectable conventional troponin T levels. Int J Cardiol 2013;168(4):3609–12.

35. Arenja N, Reichlin T, Drexler B, et al. Sensitive cardiac troponin in the diagnosis and risk stratification of acute heart failure. J Intern Med 2012;271(6):598–607.

36. Xue Y, Clopton P, Peacock WF, et al. Serial changes in high-sensitive troponin i predict outcome in patients with decompensated heart failure. Eur J Heart Fail 2011;13(1):37–42.

37. Latini R, Masson S, Anand IS, et al. Prognostic value of very low plasma concentrations of troponin T in patients with stable chronic heart failure. Circulation 2007;116(11):1242–9.

38. Grodin JL, Neale S, Wu Y, et al. Prognostic comparison of different sensitivity cardiac troponin assays in stable heart failure. Am J Med 2015;128(3):276–82.

39. Jungbauer CG, Riedlinger J, Buchner S, et al. High-sensitive troponin T in chronic heart failure correlates with severity of symptoms, left ventricular dysfunction and prognosis independently from N-terminal pro-b-type natriuretic peptide. Clin Chem Lab Med 2011;49(11):1899–906.

40. Gravning J, Askevold ET, Nymo SH, et al. Prognostic effect of high-sensitive troponin t assessment in elderly patients with chronic heart failure results from the CORONA Trial. Circ Heart Fail 2014;7(1): 96–103.

41. Nagarajan V, Hernandez AV, Tang WHW. Prognostic value of cardiac troponin in chronic stable heart failure: a systematic review. Heart 2012;98(24):1778–86.

42. Pandey A, Golwala H, Sheng S, et al. Factors associated with and prognostic implications of cardiac troponin elevation in decompensated heart failure with preserved ejection fraction. JAMA Cardiol 2016;2(2):136–45.

43. Sanders-Van Wijk S, Van Empel V, Davarzani N, et al. Circulating biomarkers of distinct pathophysiological pathways in heart failure with preserved vs. reduced left ventricular ejection fraction. Eur J Heart Fail 2015;17(10):1006–14.

44. Dengler TJ, Zimmermann R, Braun K, et al. Elevated serum concentrations of cardiac troponin T in acute allograft rejection after human heart transplantation. J Am Coll Cardiol 1998;32(2):405–12.

45. Ambrosi P, Kreitmann B, Fromonot J, et al. Plasma ultrasensitive cardiac troponin during long-term follow-up of heart transplant recipients. J Card Fail 2015;21(2):103–7.

46. Hofmann NP, Steuer C, Voss A, et al. Comprehensive bio-imaging using myocardial perfusion reserve index during cardiac magnetic resonance imaging and high-sensitive troponin T for the prediction of outcomes in heart transplant recipients. Am J Transplant 2014;14(11):2607–16.

47. Ford I, Shah ASV, Zhang R, et al. High-sensitivity cardiac troponin, statin therapy, and risk of coronary heart disease. J Am Coll Cardiol 2016; 68(25):2719–28.

48. Yancy CW, Jessup M, Bozkurt B, et al. 2016 ACC/AHA/HFSA focused update on new pharmacological therapy for heart failure: an update of the 2013 ACCF/AHA guideline for the management of heart failure. J Am Coll Cardiol 2016;68(13):1476–88.

Growth Hormone as Biomarker in Heart Failure

Alberto M. Marra, MD[a,1], Emanuele Bobbio, MD[b,1],
Roberta D'Assante, PhD[a], Andrea Salzano, MD[b,c],
Michele Arcopinto, MD[b], Eduardo Bossone, MD, PhD[d],
Antonio Cittadini, MD[b,e,*]

KEYWORDS

• Chronic heart failure • Growth hormone • IGF-1 • Anabolic deficiency • Biomarker • Outcomes

KEY POINTS

• The growth hormone (GH) and insulin growth factor 1 axis play a pivotal role in chronic heart failure (CHF).
• Both GH as well as deficiency are associated with impaired functional capacity and poor outcomes.
• GH replacement therapy represents a possible future therapeutic option in CHF.

INTRODUCTION

The neuro-hormonal model has radically changed our understanding of chronic heart failure (CHF) pathophysiology and represented the theoretic background for the implementation of landmark clinical trials, which in turn have dramatically changed the natural history of this disease.[1] This model is rooted in the ubiquitous overactivation of different molecular pathways, such as the sympathetic nervous system, renin-angiotensin-aldosterone, and cytokines' system overexpression, that maintain the heart function within a homeostatic range, after an index event.[2] However, such prolonged overactivity gradually leads to a maladaptive remodeling of the left ventricle architecture and function, with attendant impairment of exercise capacity and occurrence of poor outcomes.[2] The blockade of the sympathetic nervous system (with β-blockers) and the inhibition of the renin-angiotensin-aldosterone pathway (with angiotensin-converting enzyme [ACE] inhibitors, angiotensin receptor blockers [ARBs], and aldosterone-antagonists) constitutes the bedrock of current pharmacologic therapy for heart failure with reduced ejection fraction (HFrEF),[3,4] taking into account the associated consistent improvements in terms of morbidity and mortality granted by those pharmaceutical classes.[5] However, CHF is still burdened by high mortality (worse than that of many cancers), frequent comorbidities, and, consequently, tremendous associated health care costs.[1] For this reason, in the last decades several other pathophysiologic models were proposed to complement the paradigm of neuro-hormonal hyperactivity. More specifically, the

Disclosure Statement: The authors have nothing to disclose.
[a] IRCCS SDN, Via Gianturco, 113, 80143 Naples, Italy; [b] Department of Translational Medical Sciences, Federico II University, Via Pansini, 5, 80131 Naples, Italy; [c] Department of Cardiovascular Sciences and NIHR Biomedical Research Centre, University of Leicester, Glenfield Hospital, Groby Road LE3 9QP, Leicester, UK; [d] Heart Department, University Hospital Salerno, Via Enrico de Marinis, 84013 Cava de' Tirreni SA, Italy; [e] Interdisciplinary Research Centre in Biomedical Materials (CRIB), Via Pansini, 5, 80131 Naples, Italy
[1] These authors equally contributed to the work.
* Corresponding author. Department of Translational Medical Sciences, "Federico II" University-School of Medicine, Via Pansini 5, Naples 80131, Italy.
E-mail address: antonio.cittadini@unina.it

Heart Failure Clin 14 (2018) 65–74
http://dx.doi.org/10.1016/j.hfc.2017.08.008
1551-7136/18/© 2017 Elsevier Inc. All rights reserved.

concept is emerging that also downregulation of a portfolio of several biologically active molecules impact on heart failure progression, not the hyper-activation of the systems previously listed. In this regard, multiple anabolic deficiencies have been consistently described in HFrEF[6–8] and, more importantly, are significantly associated with several indexes of physical performance and sur-vival. Chief among these is the reduced activity of growth hormone (GH) and its tissue effector insulinlike growth factor 1 (IGF-1).[9] This review is focused on the involvement of the GH/IGF-1 axis in CHF and its possible use, either as a clinical biomarker or as a potential therapeutic target.

GROWTH HORMONE/INSULINLIKE GROWTH FACTOR 1 AXIS PHYSIOLOGY

Several biological processes require the pituitary secretion of GH. One of the main effects of the interaction between GH and its specific receptors (GHRs) is the activation of a complex signaling cascade that leads to the hepatic production of its major biological mediator IGF-I.

GH and IGF-1 are linked by a long-loop feed-back because the IGF-1 produced in the liver in response to GH inhibits GH release through the stimulation of somatostatin release.[9]

The GH/IGF-I axis is regarded as the most power-ful anabolic system in nature. Although this pivotal mechanism is still poorly understood, it is well known that the GH/IGF-I axis is responsible for post-natal growth by increasing both bone length and density and muscle mass during childhood and adolescence.[10] Moreover, it has important effects by regulating carbohydrates and lipid metabolism, the latter preferentially on visceral adipose tissue.[11] It has been documented that IGF-I is also released by several other tissues; thus, IGF-1 acts not only as classic endocrine hormone but also in an auto-crine and paracrine manner. IGF-1 circulates in blood either free or bound to specific binding pro-teins that prolong its half-life.[12] To date, 6 IGF-1 binding proteins (IGFBPs) have been identified and represent an elaborate system for regulating IGF-1 activity. In particular, almost 90% of circulating IGF-I is part of a ternary complex, also composed of IGF-specific binding protein 3 (IGFBP-III) and the acid-labile subunit.[13] This complex allows IGF-I to reach several tissues, where it binds to its own re-ceptor (IGF1R), leading to the activation of the PI3K/Akt (phosphatidylinositide 3-kinases (PI3K)/alpha serine/threonine-protein kinase [Akt]) signaling pathway, which in turn promotes cell growth, en-hances glucose transport, inhibits apoptosis, and acts along with interleukin 6 to protect cells from tu-mor necrosis factor (TNF)-α cytotoxicity.[9]

It should be noted that besides the regulation of the somatic growth, this anabolic axis has a signif-icant impact on the cardiovascular system by sup-porting cardiac growth and performance. The activation of IGF-I receptors expressed in cardio-myocytes determines a direct effect on the reduc-tion of the systemic vascular resistance by inducing the production of nitric oxide, promotes the contractility of cardiomyocytes mainly by increasing intracellular calcium concentration and calcium sensitization of the myofilaments, and preserves capillary density.[14] Of note, both GH and IGF-1 are endowed with growth-promoting properties within the myocardium and increase protein synthesis in the cardiomyocytes.[15]

IGF-1 also induces the reuptake of calcium by the sarcoplasmic reticulum by regulating the sarco/endoplasmic reticulum Ca2+-ATPase (SERCA2), which is involved in diastolic function.

Moreover, several studies performed in experi-mental models of heart failure demonstrated that GH/IGF-1 activation augments SERCA2 myocar-dial content, attenuates left ventricular remodel-ing, and enhances intracellular Akt signaling.[16] In addition, it plays a pivotal role by regulating car-diac growth, cardiomyocyte size, and metabolism by stimulating amino acid uptake for protein syn-thesis and promoting the transcription of genes specifically expressed in the cardiac muscle.[9] Of note, GH per se increases protein synthesis in the isolated perfused heart by augmenting amino acid trasport.[17]

PATHOPHYSIOLOGY OF GROWTH HORMONE/INSULINLIKE GROWTH FACTOR 1 IMPAIRMENT IN HEART FAILURE

GH deficiency (GHD) is a common finding in CHF with a prevalence ranging from 32% to 53% ac-cording to different reports.[14,18,19] IGF-1 has a remarkable positive effect on the cardiovascular system, including antiapoptotic and growth-promoting action, vasodilation and endothelial protection, and increase of cardiac contrac-tility.[9,15] Most of the studies performed in CHF reported reduced IGF-1 serum levels when compared with healthy controls.[18,20–22] IGF-1 levels were remarkably reduced in patients with advanced heart failure[23] or cachexia.[24] Many ex-planations were provided regarding the underlying mechanism of impaired GH/IGF-1 secretion in CHF. The first hypothesis is rooted in hypoperfu-sion and reduced oxygen supply, which is the typical hallmark of CHF clinical syndrome. Indeed, 25 children with GHD were evaluated with brain MRI and compared with healthy controls. In these series, pituitary stalk enhancement was significantly lower in GHD than controls, probably related to a mismatch between arterial perfusion and venous drainage.[25] The hemodynamic impairment occurring in CHF is likely to alter the local perfusion of the pituitary gland, specifically by venous drainage stasis and/or deteriorated arterial blood supply leading to cell death and consequently GHD. This speculation is not sufficient to explain alone the high GHD prevalence observed in CHF. Indeed, this theory was never proved by a neuroimaging study of the hypothalamic-pituitary axis of patients with CHF. Primary hypothalamic damage was also hypothesized by Broglio and colleagues[18] who found in their report in a CHF cohort a blunted response to different provocative tests, such as GH releasing hormone (GHRH), GHRH + arginine, and GH-related peptides. The same investigators also excluded the presence of hyperactivity of somatostatin pulse, which physiologically counteracts GH secretion.[18]

An additional central role might be also played by several other factors, albeit not completely understood. As a matter of fact, abnormalities of GH/IGF-1 secretion are likely to be found in several chronic wasting conditions characterized by inflammatory activation and cytokine overexpression.[26–28] In chronic illness, reduced hepatic synthesis of peptide hormones produced by the liver is dramatically impaired; at the same stage, a peripheral GH resistance was reported.[24] Many patients affected by CHF experience secondary pulmonary hypertension and consequent right heart failure and backward liver congestion that may also impair IGF-1 secretion.[29] Another explication might be found in background therapy for CHF. Indeed, both ACE inhibitors[30] and β-blockers[31] are likely to modify IGF-1 secretion through direct inhibitions of the IGF-1 signaling pathway.

Taken all together, it is not possible to put forward a single explanatory pathophysiologic mechanism of the occurrence of GH/IGF-1 impairment in CHF. Most probably, synergy and interaction of different molecular pathways and concomitant pharmacologic issues might represent the underpinnings of this phenomena (**Fig. 1**).

GROWTH HORMONE DEFICIENCY IN HEART FAILURE

Adult GHD is a heterogeneous disorder characterized by unspecific clinical features. It may arise during childhood or adult life, resulting from several causes, including trauma, genetic abnormalities, structural or iatrogenic lesions, and infiltrative diseases.[32]

Diagnosing GHD in adults may be challenging because of the lack of a single biological end point, such as growth failure and the pulsatile endogenous GH secretion, influenced by anthropometric factors, physical activity, and sleep patterns.[33]

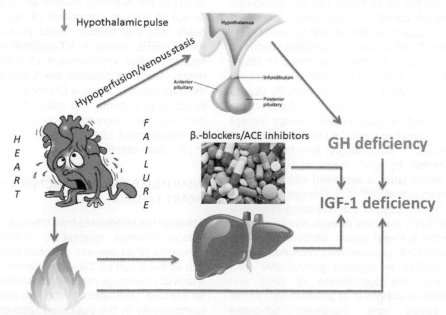

Inflammation and Cytokine overexpression

Fig. 1. Pathophysiologic background of GH/IGF-1 impairment in heart failure.

International consensus guidelines have endorsed the insulin tolerance test as the gold standard test for evaluation of adult GHD, but its safety concerns restrict its broader use in the United States.[34–36]

Because of its high discriminatory power, convenience, and reproducibility, the contemporary administration of GHRH and arginine has gained wide acceptance for GHD diagnosis,[18,37,38] in particular in patients with CHF, in whom hypoglycemia could be unsafe and should consequently be avoided.

Because the arginine potentiates the GHRH stimulatory effect by inhibiting somatostatin tone, the GHRH stimulus is significantly potentiated.[39,40] An intravenous bolus of GHRH (1 mcg/kg, maximum dose 100 mcg) is administered after an infusion of arginine (0.5 g/kg, maximum dose 30 g), and blood samples for GH measurement are obtained every 15 to 30 minutes during the next 2 hours.[41] Critical for the correct diagnosis of GHD is an accurate measurement of GH levels because the results of the tests could be influenced by the analytical method. Other molecules produced in the pituitary gland (eg, prolactin) may potentially affect the measurement cross-reacting with monoclonal antibodies usually used to limit detection to the 22-kDa GH isoform. Indeed, there are many different isomers and isoforms of circulating GH, but the 22-kDa GH variant is the most common one.[42] Several population studies reported GHD being per se associated with impaired cardiac performance, increased peripheral vascular resistance, and reduced exercise capacity[9] with a positive correlation between GHD severity and cardiac impairment.[43] Moreover, at the beginning of the 1990s, a landmark article demonstrated premature mortality due to cardiovascular disease in adults with hypopituitarism under routine replacement therapy except GH, thus, suggesting a role for GHD in cardiovascular diseases.[44] Interestingly, one-third of patients affected by CHF have a concomitant GHD, when the latter is assessed with an appropriate dynamic test.[14,18,19,45] Growing evidence supports the concept of the relevance in several features of CHF. A recent prospective work published by the authors' group, performed on 130 patients with CHF prospectively recruited undergoing a GHRH + arginine provocative test, showed that the coexistence of GHD and CHF identifies a subgroup of patients with worse clinical status and increased all-cause mortality, higher depression scores, impaired quality of life, presence of left ventricular (LV) remodeling, lower physical performance, and

increased N-terminal prohormone of brain natriuretic peptide (NT-proBNP) levels.[45] Specifically, when compared with GH-sufficient patients, patients with GHD displayed larger LV volumes with elevated wall stress as well as higher filling pressures and impairment of right ventricle function. Moreover, these patients also presented with worse cardiopulmonary performance as demonstrated by a significantly lower peak oxygen consumption per unit time (Vo_2) and reduced ventilatory efficiency.[45] GH might play an influential role also in acute heart failure exacerbation. Bhandari and colleagues[46] recently evaluated serum GH concentrations in 537 patients admitted for acute heart failure (AHF), both with HFrEF phenotype (n = 415) and with the heart failure with preserved ejection fraction (HFpEF) phenotype (n = 122). The investigators found increased GH levels in both HFrEF and HFpEF ($P<.001$ and $P = .02$, respectively) in patients who experienced one of the prespecified outcome measures (either death or readmission within 1 year).[46] GH concentrations were able to independently predict (hazard ratio 1.54, 95% confidence interval 1.19–1.99, $P = .001$) outcomes in HFrEF but not in HFpEF. In the same study, the investigators performed a further analysis aimed in comparing the usefulness of GH with NT-proBNP and the Acute Decompensated Heart Failure National Registry (ADHERE) score,[47] with regard to event prediction. Interestingly, the investigators reported that the addition of GH to the ADHERE multivariate logistic model (which in turn is composed of age, sex, urea, heart rate, and systolic blood pressure) and to the ADHERE model + NT-proBNP led to a net reclassification improvement of both the prognostic scores.[46] Despite the limitations due to the evaluation of a single GH measurement taken in unfasted patients, the article for the first time demonstrated incremental prognostic utility of the assessment of a marker of GH activity also in HF acute settings.

INSULINLIKE GROWTH FACTOR 1 IN HEART FAILURE

Although the statements from international endocrinology societies suggest to consider the 2.5 percentile of an age-sex matched normal population as the cutoff for IGF-1 deficiency,[48–53] there is a lack of consensus regarding the reference values for the CHF population, taking into account the inhomogeneity in the published reports. As shown in **Table 1**, different criteria were used in the different studies in order to define the condition of IGF-1 deficiency. According to population studies,

Table 1
Summary of studies on growth hormone/insulinlike growth factor axis as biomarker in heart failure

First Author, Year	n	Setting	Cutoffs	Main Findings
Niebauer et al,[21] 1998	52	CHF	Lowest level normal subject	There are reduced skeletal muscle function and increased TNF-α, CS/DHEA, NAdr (+49%), and Adr (+136%) in patients with low IGF-1 (<104 ng/mL).
Anker et al,[24] 2001	72	CHF	Comparison among groups; no cutoff used	Cachectic patients showed an increase of total serum GH and a decrease of GHBP compared with noncachectic patients.
Al-Obaidi et al,[57] 2001	24	CHF	Comparison among groups; no cutoff used	There are elevated IGF-1 levels in patients with NYHA class I–II but not in NYHA class III–IV.
Jankowska et al,[20] 2006	208	CHF	10th percentile of a healthy subject population	IGF-1 levels are prognostic markers of mortality in multivariable models when adjusted for established prognostic factors.
Petretta et al,[23] 2007	82	CHF	Log IGF-I/GH <3.45	Low IGF-I/GH ratio independently predicts all-cause mortality.
Andreassen et al,[59] 2009	194	CHF	Lower quartile of IGF-1	There is no relevant association between IGF-1 and baseline cardiac status or prognosis.
Watanabe et al,[58] 2010	142	CHF	Log IGF1/IGFBP3 less than median value	Low IGF-1/IGFBP3 is associated with increased rates of all-cause mortality, cardiac death, and a composite of cardiac death and rehospitalization.
Arcopinto et al,[22] 2014	207	CHF	IGF-1 ≤122 ng/mL (derived from a ROC curved analysis)	Low IGF-1 levels independently predict all-cause mortality.
Bhandari et al,[46] 2016	537	AHF	GH concentration 0.11 ng/mL for males and 1.22 ng/mL for females (based on previous population studies)	GH levels independently predicted 1-y outcome in HFrEF and increased prognostic information over the ADHERE score and NT-proBNP.
Arcopinto et al,[45] 2017	130	CHF	Positivity to GHRH + arginine test and BMI-adjusted cutoffs	Patients with GHD had impaired functional capacity, LV remodeling, RV performance, elevated NT-proBNP levels, and increased all-cause mortality.
Faxen et al,[62] 2017	164	CHF	Age-standardized scores of IGF-1	There is higher IGF-1 in HFpEF than HFpEF with similar IGF-BP 1; IGF-1 predicts mortality in HFrEF but not in HFpEF.

Abbreviations: Adr, adrenalin; BMI, body mass index; CS, cortisol; DHEA, dehydroepiandrosterone; GHBP, GH binding protein; NAdr, noradrenalin; NYHA, New York Heart Association; ROC, receiver operating characteristic; RV, right ventricle.

age should be considered as the main determinant of IGF-1 cutoff levels, whereas sex and ethnicity are both likely to play a negligible role.[48] **Table 1** summarizes the studies evaluating the GH/IGF-1 axis in cohorts of patients affected by CHF. Even if most of the studies in patients with CHF show reduced total serum IGF-1 levels, others showed normal and a few even increased circulating levels. Several factors could explain the discrepancies observed among the studies: different therapeutic and anthropometric backgrounds, inhomogeneous

disease severity, and also high assay variabilities.[54] For instance, Jankowska and co-workers[20] reported an extraordinary high IGF-1 value in their study (median values greater than 250 ng/mL in all age categories of controls). Broglio and colleagues[18,38] reported low IGF-1 levels in patients with severe LV dysfunction as well as a dulled response to GHRH. Similar results were confirmed by Anwar and colleagues[55] in an elderly population of patients hospitalized for CHF and by Kontoleon and colleagues[56] in 23 stable patients with HF.

Anker and colleagues[24] evaluated the GH/IGF-1 axis in cachectic and noncachectic patients with severe heart failure. GH levels were increased in the first group, whereas IGF-1 levels were decreased compared with noncachectic patients, who showed normal IGF-1 levels. Because the IGF-1/GH ratio was 12-fold higher in noncachectic patients than in cachectic patients, these data have introduced the concept of GH resistance, defined as high GH levels and low IGF-1 levels.[24] The same year Al-Obaidi and coworkers[57] showed that patients with CHF in New York Heart Association (NYHA) class I and II (mild to moderate symptoms) displayed an elevated IGF-1 serum concentration (P = .005 vs control subjects), whereas patients with more severe disease (NYHA classes III and IV) had values comparable with healthy controls. According to these aforementioned results,[57] one can speculate that IGF-1 increases at the initial stages of the disease in order to compensate and restore the heart function at a paraphysiologic level, afterward other factors may interfere and lead to a condition of reduced IGF-1 secretion up to a frank state of GH resistance.[24]

As mentioned earlier, the different (and increasing) use of CHF medications in the last 2 decades may have played a role for these discrepant results. Indeed, ACE inhibitors and ARBs have been shown to increase IGF-1 levels in patients with CHF,[30] and beta-blockers may exert a depressive action on the GH/IGF-1 axis.[31] A consistent body of evidences suggests that low IGF-1 levels in CHF are noteworthy for many reasons. Indeed, IGF-I deficiency is associated with greater activation in cytokines and the neurohormonal system, endothelial dysfunction, impairment of skeletal muscle performance,[21] and a worse outcome.[9,22,23,46,58] Interestingly, a landmark study performed by Jankowska and coworkers[20] showed that the number of hormonal deficiencies (IGF-1, dehydroepiandrosterone sulfate, testosterone) was an independent predictor of mortality in men with HF, leading to the speculation that anabolic deficiency has an intricate interaction and that the concomitance of more hormonal abnormalities has a detrimental synergistic action on prognosis.[20] This result was also confirmed by Arcopinto and coworkers,[22] who demonstrated that low IGF-1 levels (<122 ng/mL) independently predicted a higher mortality rate.[22] In countertrend with these aforementioned findings, Andreassen and colleagues[59] were not able to find any relevant differences in LV systolic function, NT-proBNP, or prognosis in patients with low IGF-1 levels.

Indeed, as shown by Petretta and coworkers,[23] the presence of a low IGF-1/GH ratio independently predicts outcomes in a small cohort of patients with CHF. The condition of low IGF-1 and high GH depicts the state of GH resistance, which in turn was demonstrated to be associated with cachexia,[24] a terminal stage of almost all chronic illness characterized by the spread of muscle wasting and poorer outcomes.[60] It is also worth mentioning the relationship between IGF-1 and its blood transporters in the stream flow, the so-called IGFBPs, which in turn are able to determine IGF-1 bioavailability. In this regard, Watanabe and colleagues[58] demonstrated that a low IGF-1/IGFBP3 ratio is associated with increased rates of all-cause mortality, cardiac death, and a composite of cardiac death and rehospitalization. The evaluation of IGF-BP might be helpful not only in HFrEF but also in HFpEF. Indeed, Barroso and collaborates[61] demonstrated a continuum in IGF-1/IGF-BP 7 ratio from subjects with normal diastolic function, asymptomatic LV diastolic dysfunction, and HFpEF.[61] Recently, Faxen and colleagues[62] demonstrated that patients with HFpEF displayed higher IGF-1/IGF-BP 1 when compared with HFrEF, specifically due to a higher serum IGF-1 concentration. However, in the same report, low levels of IGF-1 were associated with higher mortality in HFrEF but not in HFpEF.[62] Salzano and colleagues[63] also found lower IGF-1 and higher GHD in HFrEF than HFpEF. It is worth mentioning that it is, to date, missing a prospective study dwelling on IGF-1 levels in AHF. Taking all the evidence together, growing evidence leads to consider low IGF-1 levels in CHF not only an epiphenomenon but also a key factor mechanistically linked to CHF and its severity. IGF-1 might be useful in clinical practice for risk stratification in order to identify a cluster of patients needing a more aggressive therapy.

TREATING GROWTH HORMONE/INSULINLIKE GROWTH FACTOR 1 ABNORMALITIES IN HEART FAILURE

Apart from the identification of a high-risk population and prognostic value, the GH/IGF-1 axis might represent a possible therapeutic target in CHF.

Experimental studies in different animal models reported beneficial effects on cardiac function, peripheral vascular resistance, and survival.[64–66] Furthermore, early treatment of large myocardial infarction with GH reduces pathologic LV remodeling and improves LV function.[53] The translation of these results onto the clinical arena did not lead to unequivocal results. Although there are encouraging data coming from many preliminary openlabeled pilot studies,[67–73] 2 randomized controlled clinical trials[70,74] provided neutral results. However, a pooled meta-analysis of all study of GH in

CHF showed an increase of LV ejection fraction (LVEF) and a reduction in systemic vascular resistance.[75] Moreover, GH treatment reduced LV diastolic diameter and increases LV wall thickness, determining a positive long-term modification in cardiac morphology.[75] In another meta-analysis, treatment with GH resulted in an increase of exercise duration, maximum oxygen uptake, LVEF, cardiac output, and improvement in systemic vascular resistance and NYHA class level.[76] Several explications are likely to be possible in order to explain the inconsistent results of GH administration trials, such as different study duration, target dose, end points, and the assessment of GH status.[77] In this regard, it is worth mentioning that, also in placebo-controlled studies, those patients who consistently increased IGF-1 because of GH administration experienced a significant improvement, whereas those without IGF-1 increase did not.[70] This finding could lead to 2 conclusions. First, GH should probably be administered only in those patients with an impairment of GH/IGF-1 status. Second, GH therapy should not be administered in patients with advanced CHF, which are probably already in a GH resistance state.[24] On these premises, the authors performed a randomized single-blind controlled trial, aimed at comparing the effect of GH replacement therapy in CHF with regard to GHD status.[19] In this study, patients underwent a GHRH + arginine provocative test in order to enroll only those with a real state of GHD.[19] After 6 months, GH replacement therapy improved the quality-of-life score and increased LVEF, peak oxygen uptake, exercise duration, and flow-mediated vasodilation. On the other hand, it decreased circulating NT-proBNP levels.[19] Considering these encouraging results, the authors extended this study with a 4-year follow-up in order to assess whether these effects were sustained or tend to vanish over time.[14] After a 4-year follow-up, GH replacement therapy was still associated with LV reverse remodeling, as documented by the significant reductions of both LV end-diastolic and end-systolic volume indexes and circumferential wall stress, with an increase in LVEF.[14] With regard to cardiopulmonary performance, despite that the treatment effect did not reach statistical significance, in the GH group, peak V_{O_2} increased remarkably. Although the study was not designed for hard clinical end points, it was noteworthy that there was a marked difference in the aggregate of death and hospitalization for worsening CHF in the replacement therapy arm.[14] However, the usefulness of GH replacement therapy must still be proved in a double-blind placebo controlled trial.

FUTURE PROSPECTIVE AND SUMMARY

The relationship between hormones of cardiovascular diseases is quite complex.[14,78–80] In this intricate scenario, the impairment of GH/IGF-1 plays a crucial role in CHF. Most studies showed that patients affected by this condition display a more aggressive disease, impaired functional and exercise capacity, higher neurohormonal activation, a more pronounced LV remodeling, and poorer outcomes (mortality and hospitalization) regardless of the assessment method used (GH serum levels, GHD assessment, IGF-1 and its binding proteins measurement). Given this solid background, the authors sought to implement a prospective multicenter clinical registry aimed at investigating the impact of multiple and concomitant anabolic deficiencies (including, therefore, GH and IGF-1 assessment, testosterone, insulin resistance, thyroid, and so forth) on clinical status, exercise capacity, neurohormonal activation, LV architecture and function, quality of life, hospitalization, and mortality rate in patients affected by CHF: the Trattamento Ormonale nello Scompenso CArdiaco (TOSCA), whose preliminary results will be available within a few months.[7,81]

Interestingly, GH replacement therapy represents a fascinating future therapeutic option in CHF. Although the usefulness of GH replacement therapy in CHF must still be proven in a double-blind randomized controlled trial, these results shed new light on the potential use of GH status assessment, not only in risk stratification and prognosis but also as the target of innovative therapies, meeting all the needs of a biomarker as more close as possible to the ideal one.[82]

REFERENCES

1. Braunwald E. Heart failure. JACC Heart Fail 2013;1:1–20.
2. Hartupee J, Mann DL. Neurohormonal activation in heart failure with reduced ejection fraction. Nat Rev Cardiol 2016;14:30–8.
3. Sirico D, Salzano A, Celentani D, et al. Anti remodeling therapy: new strategies and future perspective in post-ischemic heart failure: part I. Monaldi Arch Chest Dis 2015;82(4):187–94.
4. Salzano A, Sirico D, Arcopinto M, et al. Anti remodeling therapy: new strategies and future perspective in post-ischemic heart failure. Part II. Monaldi Arch Chest Dis 2015;82(4):195–201.
5. Ponikowski P, Voors AA, Anker SD, et al. 2016 ESC guidelines for the diagnosis and treatment of acute and chronic heart failure. Eur J Heart Fail 2016;18:891–975.

6. Saccà L. Heart failure as a multiple hormonal deficiency syndrome. Circ Heart Fail 2009;2:151–6.

7. Arcopinto M, Salzano A, Ferrara F, et al. The Tosca registry: an ongoing, observational, multicenter registry for chronic heart failure. Transl Med UniSa 2016;14:21–7.

8. Cittadini A, Bossone E, Marra AM, et al. Anabolic/catabolic imbalance in chronic heart failure. Monaldi Arch Chest Dis 2010;74(2):53–6 [in Italian].

9. Arcopinto M, Bobbio E, Bossone E, et al. The GH/IGF-1 axis in chronic heart failure. Endocr Metab Immune Disord Drug Targets 2013;13:76–91.

10. Melmed S. New therapeutic agents for acromegaly. Nat Rev Endocrinol 2016;12:90–8.

11. Kargi AY, Merriam GR. Diagnosis and treatment of growth hormone deficiency in adults. Nat Rev Endocrinol 2013;9:335–45.

12. Hall K. Human somatomedin. Determination, occurrence, biological activity and purification. Acta Endocrinol Suppl (Copenh) 1972;163:1052.

13. Chishima S, Kogiso T, Matsushita N, et al. The relationship between the growth hormone/insulin-like growth factor system and the histological features of nonalcoholic fatty liver disease. Intern Med 2017;56:473–80.

14. Cittadini A, Marra AM, Arcopinto M, et al. Growth hormone replacement delays the progression of chronic heart failure combined with growth hormone deficiency: an extension of a randomized controlled single-blind study. JACC Heart Fail 2013;1:325–30.

15. Isgaard J, Arcopinto M, Karason K, et al. GH and the cardiovascular system: an update on a topic at heart. Endocrine 2015;48:25–35.

16. Cittadini A, Monti MG, Iaccarino G, et al. Adenoviral gene transfer of Akt enhances myocardial contractility and intracellular calcium handling. Gene Ther 2006;13:8–19.

17. Hjalmarson A, Isaksson O, Ahrén K. Effects of growth hormone and insulin on amino acid transport in perfused rat heart. Am J Physiol 1969; 217:1795–802.

18. Broglio F, Benso A, Gottero C, et al. Patients with dilated cardiomyopathy show reduction of the somatotroph responsiveness to GHRH both alone and combined with arginine. Eur J Endocrinol 2000; 142:157–63.

19. Cittadini A, Saldamarco L, Marra AM, et al. Growth hormone deficiency in patients with chronic heart failure and beneficial effects of its correction. J Clin Endocrinol Metab 2009;94:3329–36.

20. Jankowska EA, Biel B, Majda J, et al. Anabolic deficiency in men with chronic heart failure: prevalence and detrimental impact on survival. Circulation 2006; 114:1829–37.

21. Niebauer J, Pflaum CD, Clark AL, et al. Deficient insulin-like growth factor I in chronic heart failure predicts altered body composition, anabolic deficiency, cytokine and neurohormonal activation. J Am Coll Cardiol 1998;32:393–7.

22. Arcopinto M, Isgaard J, Marra AM, et al. IGF-1 predicts survival in chronic heart failure. Insights from the T.O.S.CA. (Trattamento Ormonale Nello Scompenso CArdiaco) registry. Int J Cardiol 2014;176: 1006–8.

23. Petretta M, Colao A, Sardu C, et al. NT-proBNP, IGF-I and survival in patients with chronic heart failure. Growth Horm IGF Res 2007;17:288–96.

24. Anker SD, Volterrani M, Pflaum CD, et al. Acquired growth hormone resistance in patients with chronic heart failure: implications for therapy with growth hormone. J Am Coll Cardiol 2001;38:443–52.

25. Wang CY, Chung HW, Cho NY, et al. Idiopathic growth hormone deficiency in the morphologically normal pituitary gland is associated with perfusion delay. Radiology 2011;258:213–21.

26. Doehner W, Rauchhaus M, Ponikowski P, et al. Impaired insulin sensitivity as an independent risk factor for mortality in patients with stable chronic heart failure. J Am Coll Cardiol 2005;46: 1019–26.

27. Marra AM, Arcopinto M, Bossone E, et al. Pulmonary arterial hypertension-related myopathy: an overview of current data and future perspectives. Nutr Metab Cardiovasc Dis 2015;25:131–9.

28. Marra AM, Arcopinto M, Salzano A, et al. Detectable interleukin-9 plasma levels are associated with impaired cardiopulmonary functional capacity and all-cause mortality in patients with chronic heart failure. Int J Cardiol 2016;209:114–7.

29. Rosenkranz S, Gibbs JS, Wachter R, et al. Left ventricular heart failure and pulmonary hypertension. Eur Heart J 2016;37:942–54.

30. Yoshida T, Tabony AM, Galvez S, et al. Molecular mechanisms and signaling pathways of angiotensin II-induced muscle wasting: potential therapeutic targets for cardiac cachexia. Int J Biochem Cell Biol 2013;45:2322–32.

31. Giustina A, Veldhuis JD. Pathophysiology of the neuroregulation of growth hormone secretion in experimental animals and the human. Endocr Rev 1998; 19:717–97.

32. Molitch ME, Clemmons DR, Malozowski S, et al, Endocrine Society. Evaluation and treatment of adult growth hormone deficiency: an Endocrine Society clinical practice guideline. J Clin Endocrinol Metab 2011;96:1587–609.

33. Yuen KCJ, Cook DM, Sahasranam P, et al. Prevalence of GH and other anterior pituitary hormone deficiencies in adults with nonsecreting pituitary microadenomas and normal serum IGF-1 levels. Clin Endocrinol (Oxf) 2008;69:292–8.

34. Sumida Y, Yonei Y, Tanaka S, et al. Lower levels of insulin-like growth factor-1 standard deviation score are associated with histological severity of

non-alcoholic fatty liver disease. Hepatol Res 2015; 45:771–81.

35. Cook DM, Yuen KC, Biller BM, et al, American Association of Clinical Endocrinologists. American Association of Clinical Endocrinologists medical guidelines for clinical practice for growth hormone use in growth hormone-deficient adults and transition patients - 2009 update: executive summary of recommendations. Endocr Pract 2009;15:580–6.

36. Gordon MB, Levy RA, Gut R, et al. Trends in growth hormone stimulation testing and growth hormone dosing in adult growth hormone deficiency patients: results from the answer program. Endocr Pract 2016;22(4):396–405.

37. Makimura H, Stanley T, Mun D, et al. The effects of central adiposity on growth hormone (GH) response to GH-releasing hormone-arginine stimulation testing in men. J Clin Endocrinol Metab 2008;93:4254–60.

38. Broglio F, Fubini A, Morello M, et al. Activity of GH/IGF-I axis in patients with dilated cardiomyopathy. Clin Endocrinol (Oxf) 1999;50:417–30.

39. Barinaga M, Bilezikjian LM, Vale WW, et al. Independent effects of growth hormone releasing factor on growth hormone release and gene transcription. Nature 1985;314(6008):279–81.

40. Alba-Roth J, Müller OA, Schopohl J, et al. Arginine stimulates growth hormone secretion by suppressing endogenous somatostatin secretion. J Clin Endocrinol Metab 1988;67:1186–9.

41. Rahim A, Toogood AA, Shalet SM. The assessment of growth hormone status in normal young adult males using a variety of provocative agents. Clin Endocrinol (Oxf) 1996;45:557–62.

42. Junnila RK, Strasburger CJ, Bidlingmaier M. Pitfalls of insulin-like growth factor-i and growth hormone assays. Endocrinol Metab Clin North Am 2015;44: 27–34.

43. Colao A, Di Somma C, Cuocolo A, et al. The severity of growth hormone deficiency correlates with the severity of cardiac impairment in 100 adult patients with hypopituitarism: an observational, case-control study. J Clin Endocrinol Metab 2004;89:5998–6004.

44. Saccà L. Growth hormone: a newcomer in cardiovascular medicine. Cardiovasc Res 1997;36:3–9.

45. Arcopinto M, Salzano A, Giallauria F, et al. Growth hormone deficiency is associated with worse cardiac function, physical performance, and outcome in chronic heart failure: insights from the T.O.S.CA. GHD study. PLoS One 2017;12(1):e0170058. Buchowski M, editor.

46. Bhandari SS, Narayan H, Jones DJ, et al. Plasma growth hormone is a strong predictor of risk at 1 year in acute heart failure. Eur J Heart Fail 2016; 18:281–9.

47. Fonarow GC, Adams KF, Abraham WT, et al, ADHERE Scientific Advisory Committee, Study Group, and Investigators. Risk stratification for in-hospital mortality in acutely decompensated heart failure: classification and regression tree analysis. JAMA 2005;293(5):572.

48. Bidlingmaier M, Friedrich N, Emeny RT, et al. Reference intervals for insulin-like growth factor-1 (igf-i) from birth to senescence: results from a multicenter study using a new automated chemiluminescence IGF-I immunoassay conforming to recent international recommendations. J Clin Endocrinol Metab 2014;99:1712–21.

49. Clemmons DR. Consensus statement on the standardization and evaluation of growth hormone and insulin-like growth factor assays. Clin Chem 2011; 57:555–9.

50. Cittadini A, Isgaard J, Monti MG, et al. Growth hormone prolongs survival in experimental postinfarction heart failure. J Am Coll Cardiol 2003;41: 2154–63.

51. Duerr RL, Huang S, Miraliakbar HR, et al. Insulin-like growth factor-1 enhances ventricular hypertrophy and function during the onset of experimental cardiac failure. J Clin Invest 1995;95:619–27.

52. Su EJ, Cioffi CL, Stefansson S, et al. Gene therapy vector-mediated expression of insulin-like growth factors protects cardiomyocytes from apoptosis and enhances neovascularization. Am J Physiol Heart Circ Physiol 2003;284:H1429–40.

53. Cittadini A, Grossman JD, Napoli R, et al. Growth hormone attenuates early left ventricular remodeling and improves cardiac function in rats with large myocardial infarction. J Am Coll Cardiol 1997;29: 1109–16.

54. Ranke MB, Osterziel KJ, Schweizer R, et al. Reference levels of insulin-like growth factor I in the serum of healthy adults: comparison of four immunoassays. Clin Chem Lab Med 2003;41:1329–34.

55. Anwar A, Gaspoz JM, Pampallona S, et al. Effect of congestive heart failure on the insulin-like growth factor-1 system. Am J Cardiol 2002;90:1402–5.

56. Kontoleon PE, Anastasiou-Nana MI, Papapetrou PD, et al. Hormonal profile in patients with congestive heart failure. Int J Cardiol 2003;87:179–83.

57. Al-Obaidi MK, Hon JKF, Stubbs PJ, et al. Plasma insulin-like growth factor-1 elevated in mild-to-moderate but not severe heart failure. Am Heart J 2001;142(6):11A–5A.

58. Watanabe S, Tamura T, Ono K, et al. Insulin-like growth factor axis (insulin-like growth factor-I/insulin-like growth factor-binding protein-3) as a prognostic predictor of heart failure: association with adiponectin. Eur J Heart Fail 2010;12: 1214–22.

59. Andreassen M, Kistorp C, Raymond I, et al. Plasma insulin-like growth factor I as predictor of progression and all cause mortality in chronic heart failure. Growth Horm IGF Res 2009;19:486–90.

60. Fülster S, Tacke M, Sandek A, et al. Muscle wasting in patients with chronic heart failure: results from the studies investigating co-morbidities aggravating heart failure (SICA-HF). Eur Heart J 2013;34:512–9.

61. Barroso MC, Kramer F, Greene SJ, et al. Serum insulin-like growth factor-1 and its binding protein-7: potential novel biomarkers for heart failure with preserved ejection fraction. BMC Cardiovasc Disord 2016;16:199.

62. Faxén UL, Hage C, Benson L, et al. HFpEF and HFrEF display different phenotypes as assessed by IGF-1 and IGFBP-1. J Card Fail 2017;23: 293–303.

63. Salzano A, Marra AM, Ferrara F, et al, T.O.S.CA. investigators. Multiple hormone deficiency syndrome in heart failure with preserved ejection fraction. Int J Cardiol 2016;225:1–3.

64. Yang R, Bunting S, Gillett N, et al. Growth hormone improves cardiac performance in experimental heart failure. Circulation 1995;92:262–7.

65. Duerr RL, McKirnan MD, Gim RD, et al. Cardiovascular effects of insulin-like growth factor-1 and growth hormone in chronic left ventricular failure in the rat. Circulation 1996;93:2188–96.

66. Ryoke T, Gu Y, Mao L, et al. Progressive cardiac dysfunction and fibrosis in the cardiomyopathic hamster and effects of growth hormone and angiotensin-converting enzyme inhibition. Circulation 1999;100:1734–43.

67. Fazio S, Sabatini D, Capaldo B, et al. A preliminary study of growth hormone in the treatment of dilated cardiomyopathy. N Engl J Med 1996;334:809–14.

68. Genth-Zotz S, Zotz R, Geil S, et al. Recombinant growth hormone therapy in patients with ischemic cardiomyopathy: effects on hemodynamics, left ventricular function, and cardiopulmonary exercise capacity. Circulation 1999;99(1):18–21.

69. Spallarossa P, Rossettin P, Minuto F, et al. Evaluation of growth hormone administration in patients with chronic heart failure secondary to coronary artery disease. Am J Cardiol 1999;84:430–3.

70. Perrot A, Ranke MB, Dietz R, et al. Growth hormone treatment in dilated cardiomyopathy. J Card Surg 2001;16(2):127–31.

71. Napoli R, Guardasole V, Matarazzo M, et al. Growth hormone corrects vascular dysfunction in patients with chronic heart failure. J Am Coll Cardiol 2002; 39:90–5.

72. Acevedo M, Corbalán R, Chamorro G, et al. Administration of growth hormone to patients with advanced cardiac heart failure: effects upon left ventricular function, exercise capacity, and neurohormonal status. Int J Cardiol 2003;87:185–91.

73. Fazio S, Palmieri EA, Affuso F, et al. Effects of growth hormone on exercise capacity and cardiopulmonary performance in patients with chronic heart failure. J Clin Endocrinol Metab 2007;92:4218–23.

74. Isgaard J, Bergh CH, Caidahl K, et al. A placebo-controlled study of growth hormone in patients with congestive heart failure. Eur Heart J 1998;19: 1704–11.

75. Le Corvoisier P, Hittinger L, Chanson P, et al. Cardiac effects of growth hormone treatment in chronic heart failure: a meta-analysis. J Clin Endocrinol Metab 2007;92:180–5.

76. Tritos NA, Danias PG. Growth hormone therapy in congestive heart failure due to left ventricular systolic dysfunction: a meta-analysis. Endocr Pract 2008;14:40–9.

77. Arcopinto M, Salzano A, Isgaard J, et al. Hormone replacement therapy in heart failure. Curr Opin Cardiol 2015;30:277–84.

78. Pasquali D, Arcopinto M, Renzullo A, et al. Cardiovascular abnormalities in Klinefelter syndrome. Int J Cardiol 2013;168:754–9.

79. Marra AM, Arcopinto M, Bobbio E, et al. An unusual case of dilated cardiomyopathy associated with partial hypopituitarism. Intern Emerg Med 2012;7:85–7.

80. Salzano A, Arcopinto M, Marra AM, et al. Klinefelter syndrome, cardiovascular system, and thromboembolic disease: review of literature and clinical perspectives. Eur J Endocrinol 2016;175:R27–40.

81. Bossone E, Limongelli G, Malizia G, et al. The T.O.S.CA. project: research, education and care. Monaldi Arch Chest Dis 2015;76(4):198–203.

82. Ahmad T, Fiuzat M, Felker GM, et al. Novel biomarkers in chronic heart failure. Nat Rev Cardiol 2012;9:347–59.

Galectin-3 in Heart Failure
An Update of the Last 3 Years

Carolin Gehlken, MD, Navin Suthahar, MD,
Wouter C. Meijers, MD, PhD, FHFA,
Rudolf A. de Boer, MD, PhD, FESC, FHFA*

KEYWORDS

- Galectin-3 • Heart failure • Fibrosis • Galectin-3 inhibitor • Biomarker • Prognosis

KEY POINTS

- Galectin-3 is a pleiotropic protein that is produced after organ injury and secreted in the systemic circulation.
- Galectin-3 is an established biomarker and, in a recent meta-analysis comprising 32,350 participants with a total of 323090 person-years of follow-up, galectin-3 was associated with all-cause and cardiovascular mortality.
- Galectin-3 is a protein with important biological functions, especially fibrosis formation, and as such is currently explored as a potential target for therapy.

INTRODUCTION

This article provides an update regarding the most recent published literature on galectin-3 as a biomarker in heart failure (HF) and gives an outlook toward its use as a biotarget.[1] In the last decade, several reviews from our group and others have summarized the articles on galectin-3 as an HF biomarker.[2–8] The authors have included articles extracted from the PubMed library up to April 2017.

HF is an important cause of morbidity and mortality in the Western world and approximately 10% of the people more than 70 years of age are diagnosed with HF.[9] Despite considerable advances in diagnosis and management of HF, 5-year mortality still remains around 50%, which is extremely high. The prevalence of HF is globally increasing, mainly because of the aging population[10] and increased success rates in treating cardiovascular diseases that precede HF, including myocardial infarction (MI) and hypertension.

HF is also an expensive disorder, often requiring periods of hospitalization, and this adds significantly to the burden of disease. According to an estimation, the annual cost of HF in the United States will increase from US$31 billion to US$70 billion by 2030.[11] Therefore, avoiding unnecessary HF hospitalizations is a top priority in HF management.

Patients with HF usually present with the clinical symptoms of fatigue, as well as shortness of breath and peripheral edema, which result from insufficient cardiac function. The authors use the term HF for the early stage of the disease even when clinical symptoms may not yet be present. According to the 2016 European Society of Cardiology (ESC) guidelines, HF is classified as either HF with preserved ejection fraction (HFpEF; ie, EF ≥ 50%), HF with midrange ejection fraction

Conflicts of Interest: None declared.
Department of Cardiology, University of Groningen, University Medical Center Groningen, PO Box 30.001, Groningen 9700 RB, The Netherlands
* Corresponding author.
E-mail address: r.a.de.boer@umcg.nl

Heart Failure Clin 14 (2018) 75–92
http://dx.doi.org/10.1016/j.hfc.2017.08.009
1551-7136/18/© 2017 Elsevier Inc. All rights reserved.

(HFmrEF; EF 40%–49%), and HF with reduced ejection fraction (HFrEF; EF<40%).[12] Different underlying disorders lead to the development of HF, as described elsewhere.[12–14]

Biomarkers reflect pathophysiologic mechanisms occurring in the body and are usually used as adjuncts in patient management. As such, biomarkers may find their utility in HF diagnosis, prognosis, and risk stratification; although their use in HF has expanded rapidly, several biomarkers have still not made their way into regular patient management. Current HF guidelines focus primarily on B-type natriuretic peptide (BNP) or its biologically inert amino-terminal pro-peptide, N-terminal proBNP (NT-proBNP).[12] However, NT-proBNP usage has limitations: Although NT-proBNP levels can be used to diagnose both types of HF, low levels might not exclude HFpEF diagnosis.[15]

The 2013 American College of Cardiology Foundation/American Heart Association guideline for the management of HF recommends the use of galectin-3 for risk stratification as well as for prognosis in patients with moderate and severe HF (class IIb).[16] Although current ESC guidelines on HF do not recommend galectin-3 for clinical practice, it seems to be a useful biomarker in various settings, which are discussed later.

Galectin-3 is one of 14 members of the lectin family and is encoded by a single gene (LGALS3); it binds various β-galactosides using its carbohydrate recognition domain (CRD), and elicits several biological effects. The CRD consists of approximately 130 amino acids and is indicated in the pathophysiology of HF. Galectin-3 also plays an important role in inflammation; tissue repair, including fibrogenesis; as well as cardiac ventricular remodeling, which is an important hallmark in HF[2,14,17] (**Fig. 1**).

This article discusses the utility of galectin-3 in new-onset, acute, and chronic HF, including HFrEF and HFpEF. First, it highlights different diagnostic assays and reference ranges of galectin-3 in various populations.

GALECTIN-3 ASSAYS

Establishing a reproducible and accurate method to measure galectin-3 in the circulation is important for research as well as in clinics and there are several commercial galectin-3 assays that provide an accurate measurement of circulating galectin-3. The most commonly used galectin-3 assays are summarized in **Table 1**. These assays can be used to detect galectin-3 from venous blood samples, which can be collected in EDTA (ethylenediaminetetraacetic acid) tubes or in serum. After separation, the serum or plasma may be stored at −70°C for approximately 10 years and can undergo up to 9 freeze-thaw cycles without significantly influencing galectin-3 test results.[18] The BG Medicine (BGM) galectin-3 enzyme-linked immunosorbent assay (ELISA) kit and R&D ELISA kit are manual assays, whereas

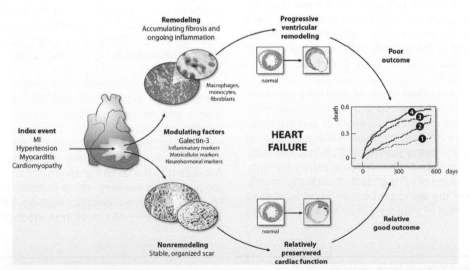

Fig. 1. Mechanism underlying HF. An index event such as a MI, endocarditis, or long-standing hypertension causes stress to the heart. This index event provokes a release of different cytokines that may cause a pathologic remodeling with an upregulation in fibrosis and inflammation; on-going pathologic remodeling leads to a poor outcome with an increased mortality. In contrast, there can be a nonremodeling with a stable and organized scar and a relatively preserved cardiac function. (*From* de Boer RA, Meissner M, van Veldhuisen DJ. Galectin-3. In: Maisel AS, editor. New Delhi (India): Jaypee Brothers, 2012. p. 206; with permission.)

Galectin-3 in Heart Failure

Table 1
Comparison of galectin-3 assays

	Sample Volume (µL)	Duration (h)	Total Imprecisions Intravariability In CV (%)	Intervariability In CV (%)	Detection Limit LoB (ng/mL)	LoD (ng/mL)	LoQ (ng/mL)	Measuring Range (ng/mL)	Interference	Cross Reactivity	Percentiles[d]		
BGM	30	3.5	3.2	5.6	0.86	1.13	1.32	1.4–94.8	b	c	19	22.1	26.2
ARCHITECT: Stat	25[a]	18	3.4	4.1	0.8	1	4	4–114	b	c	22.4	25.7	27.5
ARCHITECT: Routine	25[a]	28	4.1	4.9	0.8	1	4	4–114	b	c	22.4	25.7	27.5
VIDAS	200	20	1.3	5.5	2.2	2.4	3.3	3.3–100	b	c	—	—	—
R and D	50	4.5	3.9	5.9	—	0.02	—	0.313–10	b	c	9.1	9.9	10.6
Alere	10	—	12	5	—	—	—	0.5–86.2	b	c	—	—	—

Abbreviations: BGM, BG Medicine; CV, cardiovascular; LoB, limit of blank; LoD, limit of detection; LoQ, limit of quantification.
[a] Plus 50 µL of dead volume.
[b] No interference with conjugated bilirubin; unconjugated bilirubin; lipidemia; triglycerides; bovine serum albumin; cholesterol; creatinine; hemoglobin; galectins 1, 2, 4, 7, 8, 9, 10, 14; MAC-2BP and commonly used cardiovascular medication. Interference with hemolyzed samples, human antimouse antibody, rheumatoid factor, and verapamil.
[c] No cross reactivity with collagens I, III, and 9, and other galectins.
[d] Percentiles based on general population.

From Meijers WC, van der Velde AR, de Boer RA. The ARCHITECT galectin-3 assay: comparison with other automated and manual assays for the measurement of circulating galectin-3 levels in heart failure. Expert Rev Mol Diagn 2014;4:262; with permission.

ARCHITECT and VIDAS are the frequently used automated assays (using the same antibodies as BGM assay).

BGM developed a galectin-3 ELISA kit and used rat monoclonal antimouse galectin-3 antibody attached to a microtiter plate. The secondary antibody is a traced mouse monoclonal antihuman galectin-3 antibody. The concentration of galectin-3 can be determined with spectrophotometry with the help of another substrate, and at least 30 μL of serum or plasma is required. This assay is not automated, and has a long turnaround time of 3.5 hours; however, it is often used because of its low operating costs, and because it has received US Food and Drug Administration (FDA) approval.[18–20] The R&D ELISA uses the same sandwich ELISA technique as BGM, but requires a sample volume of 50 μl; it is not FDA approved and is mainly used in research settings.[18,21]

A cooperation of BGM and Abbott provided the first automated galectin-3 assay, known as ARCHITECT. The ARCHITECT assay uses the same antibodies as the BGM galectin-3 ELISA kit. In addition, a tracer as well as another substrate is required to run a chemiluminescent immunoassay. Abbott offers 2 different demand-adapted assays and both these assays require a 25-μL sample volume. It has a short turnaround time of only 18 minutes, and therefore can be effective when multiple samples are analyzed on a daily basis.[18,22,23] The VIDAS, produced by bioMérieux, is another automated immunoassay based on a strip system, which can be evaluated using a specific machine. Although this assay requires a high sample volume of 200 μL, it has a short runtime of 20 minutes. VIDAS is consistent with the BGM assay; however, it has higher running costs.[18,24]

In order to interpret the information conferred by changes in biomarker levels over time, it is of crucial importance to understand parameters of variation. A recent study investigated the variation of common and novel biomarkers in 28 healthy controls and 83 patients with HF. Galectin-3 was found to be a stable biomarker with very low variability. The intraindividual coefficient of variation (CVi) was reported, as well as the reference change value (RCV), which is a marker of percentage of change that indicates a relevant change. Galectin-3 had low indices of variation: a CVi of 8.1% and an RCV of 25.0%, which is lower than, for example, NT-proBNP (CVi, 16.6% and RCV, 64.3%).[25] A low CVi of galectin-3 (short-term, 4.5%; long-term, 5.5%) was also shown in 20 healthy controls and 59 patients with HF.[26]

GALECTIN-3 LEVELS: TRENDS IN HEALTHY INDIVIDUALS

Galectin-3 reference intervals in healthy individuals have been derived from large cohort studies, such as the prevention of renal and vascular end-stage disease (PREVEND) study, Framingham study, and the National FINRISK study. Galectin-3 levels gradually increase with age[23,27] and are also slightly higher in women than in men.[27] Galectin-3 levels also vary depending on race. In a substudy of the Atherosclerosis Risk in Communities (ARIC) study, galectin-3 levels were evaluated in 1809 subjects; although baseline levels were higher in healthy black individuals compared with healthy white individuals, galectin-3 did not strongly predict HF and death in black people. However, galectin-3 levels were independently associated with HF or death as a composite end point and also provided improved discrimination in Harrel's C statistic in white subjects.[28]

NEW-ONSET HEART FAILURE

New-onset HF may present as acutely decompensated HF (ADHF; eg, after acute MI) or may start subacutely, which makes the diagnosis of the condition more difficult; for example, in dilated cardiomyopathy.[12] The following studies highlight the use of galectin-3 as a biomarker in predicting new-onset HF in the general population.

In the Framingham Offspring Cohort, which included 3353 participants (initially N = 3450), galectin-3 was significantly associated with an increased risk for new-onset HF and all-cause mortality after adjustment for BNP and several other clinical variables.[29] The Rancho Bernardo Study was an outcome analysis of 1389 subjects from the general elderly population with a mean age of 70 years. Increased galectin-3 was a proportional predictor of cardiovascular death and all-cause mortality, also after adjustment for NT-proBNP, in subjects without previously diagnosed cardiovascular disease.[30] However, this study did not evaluate new-onset HF.

The FINRISK cohort (N = 8444) study showed that increased galectin-3 levels were proportional to an increased risk of cardiovascular events in the general population. However, there was no significant relationship in predicting HF incidence after adjusting for NT-proBNP.[31] In addition, in the PREVEND cohort study (N = 5958), which evaluated the usefulness of serial galectin-3 measurements in the general population, a persistently increased galectin-3 level independently showed an increased risk of developing new-onset HF.[32]

A recently published meta-analysis including 18 studies with 32,350 subjects showed an increased risk of all-cause mortality, cardiovascular mortality, as well as HF in individuals with increased galectin-3 levels.[1] The utility of galectin-3 levels to predict all-cause mortality and new-onset HF in the general population is summarized in **Table 2**.

PROGNOSIS AND RISK STRATIFICATION: ACUTE HEART FAILURE

Acute HF (AHF) is characterized by a sudden onset of HF symptoms, usually also combined with signs of HF.[12] AHF can be a new-onset HF, or, more commonly, a decompensation of preexisting HF (chronic HF [CHF]), and can be caused by intrinsic or extrinsic factors, which are described elsewhere.[12] AHF is the leading cause of hospitalization in elderly people in Europe, and is a major contributor to overall health care cost as well as mortality.[33]

Although galectin-3 levels are usually increased in patients with AHF, it has a limited role in diagnosing AHF.[34] BNP, a marker of myocardial stretch and overload, is the leading biomarker in diagnosing AHF in patients presenting with dyspnea to the emergency department.[35] Because galectin-3 is a slow marker, reflecting fibrotic processes, it seems to be a particularly useful in identifying patients with AHF who are at an increased risk for future events and in selecting those who require a more intensive follow-up. Several studies have been published and reviewed demonstrating the utility of galectin-3 in AHF.[36–41]

In 2010, a subanalysis conducted on 56 patients with ADHF showed a significant relationship between increased galectin-3 levels and increase in 4-year mortality, independent of echocardiographic parameters.[34]

More recently, Mueller and colleagues[35] included 251 subjects with AHF and considered galectin-3 useful in determining the probability of 1-year all-cause mortality; soluble suppressor of tumorgenicity 2 (sST2) and BNP were also equally useful in predicting this end point. Another study, including 101 patients, showed a significant improvement in predicting the likelihood of a 60-day readmission in patients with ADHF if galectin-3 was evaluated together with BNP. When used as a sole marker, galectin-3 also

Table 2
Galectin-3 in the general population

Study or Author Name, Date	Sample Size (N)	Assay	Median Gal-3 Levels (ng/mL)	Follow-up Period (y)	End Points	Main Findings/ Results
Framingham Offspring Cohort,[29] 2012	3353	BGM	Women, 14.3 Men, 13.1	8.1	Several sequences of events	Galectin-3 significantly predicted new-onset HF after adjustment for BNP and several other clinical variables in general population
FINRISK cohort,[31] 2015	8444	ARCHITECT Galectin-3	Women, 12.0 Men, 11.5	15	All-cause mortality Cardiac death MI Ischemic stroke HF	Predictor for incident HF and death after correction for NT-proBNP in general population
PREVEND study,[78] 2016	5958	BGM	Baseline, 10.7; after ~9 y, 11.5	Median 9.3	New-onset HF CV death All-cause mortality New-onset atrial fibrillation CV event	Increases in galectin-3 associated with increased blood pressure and urinary albumin >30 mg/24 h

Abbreviations: BGM, BG Medicine; BNP, B-type natriuretic peptide; CV, cardiovascular; Gal-3, galectin-3; HF, heart failure; MI, myocardial infarction; NT-proBNP, N-terminal proBNP.

showed significant prognostic value in predicting 60-day readmission in patients with ADHF with preserved ejection fraction (area under the curve, 0.85; *P*<.001).[42] Likewise, the GALectin-3 in Acute heart failure (GALA) study, which used a small study group of 115 patients, compared the values of galectin-3, NT-proBNP, and cardiac troponin I (cTnI) in predicting 30-day all-cause mortality and 1-year mortality (among other end points) and concluded that galectin-3 (but not NT-proBNP) was useful in predicting the 30-day all-cause mortality after hospital admission for AHF. The study also showed that although galectin-3 had no prognostic utility in predicting 1-year mortality, NT-proBNP had a significant predictive value; In contrast, cTnI could predict neither the 30-day nor the 1-year mortality.[43]

All the studies mentioned earlier are also in line with a pooled analysis of 902 patients hospitalized with AHF, which showed that when plasma galectin-3 levels exceeded 17.8 ng/mL, the risk for readmission (at 30, 60, 90, or 120 days) and death were significantly increased, also after adjustment for common variables, including BNP (**Fig. 2**, **Table 3**).[44] Galectin-3 very strongly reclassified patients from low-risk to high-risk categories, and vice versa; that is, patients who were classified as having high risk in fact had low risk for death and/or hospitalization. In a subsequent study, low galectin-3 levels in patients with AHF proved to be potentially effective in identifying those who could be (safely) discharged. In 592 patients in the Coordinating Study Evaluating Outcomes of Advising and Counselling in Heart Failure (COACH), galectin-3 was an effective marker in predicting the absolute absence of events within 180 days from the time of discharge after an episode of ADHF. Galectin-3 showed a

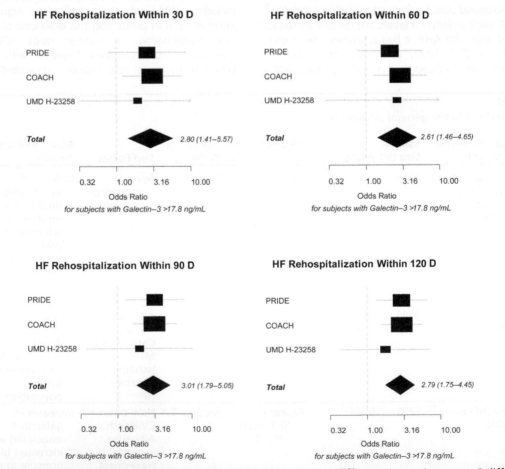

Fig. 2. Meijers pooled analysis. The odds ratio of HF rehospitalization at different time points across 3 different studies (N-terminal pro- BNP Investigation of Dyspnea in the Emergency Department [PRIDE], Coordinating Study Evaluating Outcomes of Advising and Counseling in Heart Failure [COACH], and University of Maryland [UMD] Pro-BNP for Diagnosis and Prognosis in Patients Presenting with Dyspnea study H-23258). (*From* Meijers WC, Januzzi JL, defilippi C, et al. Elevated plasma galectin-3 is associated with near-term rehospitalization in heart failure: a pooled analysis of 3 clinical trials. Am Heart J 2014;167(6):856; with permission.)

Table 3
Galectin-3 in acute heart failure studies

Study or Author Name, Date	Sample Size (N)	Assay	Median Gal-3 Levels (ng/mL)	Follow-up Period	End Points	Main Findings/Results
Subset of PRIDE study,[34] 2010	56	BGM	15	4 y	Mortality	Increased Gal-3 associated with increase in 4-y mortality, independent of echocardiographic results
Mueller et al,[35] 2016	251	ARCHITECT	22	1 y	All-cause mortality	Predictor of 1-y all-cause mortality Not useful for diagnosis of acute HF in contrast with BNP
Sudharshan et al,[42] 2017	101	BGM/Abbott Gal-3 assay	Not readmitted after 60 d 21.0/24.6 Readmitted 60 d 27.2/32.6	60 d	30-d and 60-d hospital readmission	Predicting 60-d (not 30-d) readmission in patients with HFpEF (significant without BNP)
GALA study,[43] 2017	115	VIDAS Gal-3	Patient who died, 44 Other, 26	1 y	30-d all-cause mortality	Predictor of mortality 1 mo after hospital admission
Pooled analysis of: COACH PRIDE UMD H-23258,[44] 2014	902	BGM	18.2	≥120 d	All-cause mortality and rehospitalization	Predictor for near-term readmission
COACH,[36] 2015	592	BGM	No event, 18.9 Event: 24.5	180 d	All-cause mortality and/or HF rehospitalization	Predictor of absence of events within 180 d at the time of discharge after an episode of acutely decompensated HF
RELAX-AHF trial,[45] 2017	1161	BGM	Baseline, 21.1 At 180 d, 20.6	180 d	Time to CV mortality	Gal-3: stable over time (baseline to day 60) No benefit of repeated measurements could be proved Gal-3 is not independently associated with CV mortality within 180 d
Boulogne et al,[66] 2017	55 acute HFrEF 20 chronic HFrEF	ARCHITECT	Baseline AHF, 22.8 CHF, 13.0 30 d after discharge	1 y	Death Unplanned admission for CV cause	Gal-3 level was significantly higher in AHF compared with CHF Gal-3 values remained stable in both groups over time

Abbreviations: BGM, BG medicine; BNP, B-type natriuretic peptide; CHF, chronic heart failure; COACH, coordinating study evaluating outcomes of advising and counseling in heart failure; CV, cardiovascular; Gal-3, galectin-3; GALA, GALectin-3 in Acute HF; HF, heart failure; HFpEF, HF with preserved ejection fraction; HFrEF, HF with reduced ejection fraction; PRIDE, N-terminal pro- BNP investigation of dyspnea in the emergency department; RELAX-AHF, RELAXin acute heart failure (RELAX-AHF); UMD, university of maryland Pro-BNP for Diagnosis and Prognosis in Patients Presenting with Dyspnea study H-23258.

good sensitivity in predicting the absence of events when values were less than 11.8 ng/mL. The results were also validated in the independent TRIple pill vs Usual care Management for Patients with mild-to-moderate Hypertension (TRIUMPH) HF cohort, which included 285 subjects.[36] Galectin-3 may thus be used to direct scarce resources to those patients who truly have an increased risk of having events during follow-up, and steering unnecessary care away from low-risk patients.

In contrast, some other studies showed a limited value of galectin-3 in predicting outcomes in patients with AHF. The RELAXin in Acute Heart Failure (RELAX-AHF) trial compared different biomarkers at multiple times in patients with AHF (n = 1161). Galectin-3 was stable over time (baseline to day 60) and a benefit of repeated measurements could not be proved,[45] whereas high-sensitivity C-reactive protein and sST2 had an improved predictive value on day 14 after hospital admission.[45] This finding was confirmed in a recent study involving 2033 patients with AHF from the ProB- NP Outpatient Tailored Chronic Heart Failure (PROTECT) study; galectin-3 levels remained stable over time and serial measurements offered limited prognostic value in these patients.[46]

In conclusion, plasma galectin-3 seems to be an additional risk marker in the diagnosis and prognosis of AHF. However, it is important to realize that galectin-3 is not a cardiac-specific biomarker and may also reflect other systemic pathophysiologic processes, such as activation of the inflammatory axis on top of cardiovascular disorder.

PROGNOSIS AND RISK STRATIFICATION: CHRONIC HEART FAILURE

After the initial emergency of AHF has resolved, and the condition of HF persists for more than 3 months,[47] the condition is then referred to as CHF. Like AHF, CHF may have different causes, including a diseased myocardium, abnormal loading conditions, and arrhythmias.[12] Compared healthy individuals, galectin-3 levels are usually increased in patients with CHF (Table 4).[25,46,48,49,53,54] The prognostic utility of galectin-3 in CHF was first reported in a study by Lin and colleagues[50] on 106 patients with CHF. Galectin-3 levels also correlated with markers of cardiac remodeling after adjustment for age, gender, and New York Heart Association (NYHA) class. Another study, in 2010, also showed the association between galectin-3 and left ventricular remodeling and indicated that galectin-3 was able to predict long-term all-cause mortality in

patients with CHF even after adjusting for age, gender, severity of HF, and renal function.[51]

A role for serial galectin-3 measurements in patients with CHF has also been explored. Serial galectin-3 measurements in the Valsartan Heart Failure Trial (Val-HeFT)[49] were prognostically significant in patients with CHF. Galectin-3 measurements from 1650 patients were included at the baseline, and an elevation of galectin-3 after 4 months (N = 1346) significantly correlated with HF hospitalization, all-cause mortality, and first morbid event after adjusting for NT-proBNP and estimated glomerular filtration rate (eGFR). Furthermore, there was a decrease in HF hospitalization when baseline galectin-3 levels were lower than 16.2 ng/mL.[49]

In a recent study involving patients with CHF from the Controlled Rosuvastatin Multinational Trial in Heart Failure (CORONA) (N = 1329), galectin-3 levels were measured at baseline and at 3 months; the primary composite end point was all-cause mortality or rehospitalization. Serial galectin-3 measurements were also useful in this study: a 15% increase over 3 to 6 months affords a 50% increase in death and HF rehospitalization.[52]

In contrast, previous studies showed that there was no added value of repeated galectin-3 measurements (at baseline and after 6 months) in patients with CHF.[53] Several other studies support these observations; for instance, in a recent study, serial galectin-3 measurements in 180 patients with CHF with reduced ejection fraction (EF) over 2 years did not have any significant prognostic value in predicting risk of death or cardiac transplant after adjusting for clinical variables, BNP, and cTnT.[54]

Galectin-3 levels in CHF also seem to vary depending on other factors, such as rehabilitation or comorbidities. Cardiac rehabilitation seems to reduce galectin-3 levels in patients with CHF. A recent study showed that there was a 6.3% median decrease of galectin-3 and other cardiac biomarkers, such as sST2 and midregional pro–atrial natriuretic peptide (proANP), in patients with CHF and reduced EF (ie, EF ≤ 45%) following a cardiac rehabilitation.[55] Kidney function seems to play a key role in determining serum galectin-3 values and also influences its predictive value in HF.[56–58] A Danish research group found a relationship between an increased galectin-3 plasma concentration (>16.90 ng/mL) and a reduced eGFR, along with increased levels of proANP, chromogranin A, and copeptin, in a prospective study involving 132 patients with chronic HFrEF.[58] In patients with both HF and reduced renal function, galectin-3 has a decreased predictive value after adjustment for renal function.[56] Another study

Table 4
Galectin-3 in chronic heart failure studies

Study or Author Name, Date	Sample Size (N)	Assay	Median Gal-3 Levels (ng/mL)	Follow-up Period	End Points	Main Findings/Results
Meijers et al,[25] 2017	Healthy controls = 28 CHF = 83	BGM	Controls, 10.7 CHF, 16.1	4 mo and 6 wk Up to 5 y	HF rehospitalization or all-cause mortality	Stable biomarker with very low variability
Substudy of COACH trial,[53] 2011	592	BGM	HFrEF, LVEF ≤ 40% = 19.9 HFpEF, LVEF>40% = 20.2	18 mo	Rehospitalization for HF or death	No added value of repeated galectin-3 measurements at baseline and after 6 mo in patients with HF Stronger predictive value in HFpEF Doubling of Gal-3 associated with a hazard ratio of 1.38 for primary end point after correction
Miller et al,[54] 2016	180 (LVEF ≤ 40%)	BGM	Baseline, 23.2	2 y	Death/cardiac transplant, HF-related hospitalization	Galectin-3 (>22.1 ng/mL) was predictive of the end points, but only sST2 was an independent predictor
PROTECT trial,[46] 2016	2033	Not standardized	Baseline, 36.3	180 d	30-d all-cause mortality, 30-d death or rehospitalization for renal/CV causes 180-d all-cause mortality	Stable concentration in patients with CHF who were hospitalized for AHF
Valsartan Heart Failure Trial,[49] 2013	1650	BGM	Baseline Average, 16.2 Patients who died, 18.3 Survivors, 15.8	Median, 23 mo	Mortality, first morbid event, hospitalization for HF	Increase in galectin-3 values over time was an independent predictor of worse outcome Valsartan in patients with low galectin-3 level was associated with a reduced rate of hospitalization for HF

(continued on next page)

Table 4
(continued)

Study or Author Name, Date	Sample Size (N)	Assay	Median Gal-3 Levels (ng/mL)	Follow-up Period	End Points	Main Findings/Results
Billebeau et al,[55] 2017	107 LVEF ≤ 45%	ARCHITECT	Baseline, 18.4 After CR, 17.5 No change in no-CR group (P = .595)	4-6 mo	—	Significant (P<.0001) decrease after CR
Stoltze Gaborit et al,[58] 2016	132 HFrEF	BGM	Baseline, 16.9	Cross-sectional study without follow-up	—	>16.90 ng/mL was related to a reduced eGFR and increased proANP, chromogranin A, and copeptin Galectin-3 values were not associated with echocardiographic parameters
Zamora et al,[56] 2014	876	VIDAS	12.3 for eGFR ≥ 60 mL/min/1.73 m² 16.1 for eGFR 30 to <60 mL/min/1.73 m² 24.5 for eGFR <30 mL/min/1.73 m²	Mean, 4.2 y	All-cause mortality, CV mortality, HF hospitalization	Limited value (not significant) in HF prognosis for all-cause and CV mortality after adjustment for renal function
Imran et al,[1] 2017	32,350 Meta-analysis of 18 studies, general population and patients with HF	Most commonly BGM ARCHITECT	—	Median, 5 y	CV mortality, all-cause mortality, HF	Increased values are a predictor for all-cause mortality, CV mortality, and HF
HF-ACTION trial,[59] 2014	813	BGM	Baseline, 13.9	2.5 y	All-cause mortality and all-cause hospitalization	Contributed to net risk classification of SCD when added to NT-proBNP measurements

Abbreviations: AHF, acute heartfailure; BGM, BG medicine; BNP, B-type natriuretic peptide; CHF, chronic heart failure; COACH, coordinating study evaluating outcomes of advising and counseling in heart failure; CR, cardiac rehabilitation; CV, cardiovascular; eGFR, estimated glomerular filtration rate; Gal-3, galectin-3; HF, heart failure; HF-ACTION trial, HF- a controlled trial investigating outcomes of exercise training; HFpEF, HF with preserved ejection fraction; HFrEF, HF with reduced ejection fraction; LVEF, left ventricular ejection fraction; NT-proBNP, N-terminal pro- BNP; pro-ANP, pro-atrial natriuretic peptide; SCD, sudden cardiac death; sST2, soluble suppressor of tumorgenicity 2.

involving 876 patients also showed limited value in HF prognosis when adjusted for renal function.[56]

Galectin-3 seems to add prognostic information on top of existing HF biomarkers in patients with CHF; galectin-3 and ST2 significantly contributed to net risk classification of sudden cardiac death (SCD) but not pump failure when added to NT-proBNP measurements in 813 subjects with CHF from the HF- A Controlled Trial Investigating Outcomes of Exercise Training (HF-ACTION); In contrast, NT-proBNP was a very strong predictor of deaths caused by pump failure.[59] Certain studies also indicated that the biomarker sST2 could be superior to galectin-3 in risk stratification of patients with CHF.[60] A recent study compared the utility of serial sST2 measurements with galectin-3 measurements in ambulatory patients with CHF and concluded that, in multivariable models adjusted for BNP, cTnT, and clinical variables, serial galectin-3 measurements did not reclassify patients into higher risk groups, whereas serial measurement of sST2 offered additional prognostic value in predicting death or cardiac transplant in patients with CHF.[54]

In addition, a published meta-analysis in 2017[1] showed a significant increase of cardiovascular disease mortality risk for every standard deviation increase of galectin-3 in patients with HF (hazard ratio, 1.44 [1.09–1.79]). Galectin-3 could thus provide additional prognostic value compared with that provided by conventional cardiovascular disease risk factors.

GALECTIN-3 AND HEART FAILURE WITH PRESERVED EJECTION FRACTION

Preventive medicine is becoming a major focus in modern therapy guidelines. A major part of the population more than 65 years of age is diagnosed with arterial hypertension, which can potentially lead to HFpEF. Individuals who are at a higher risk of developing HFpEF need to be identified, and galectin-3 can be an effective biomarker in early detection of HFpEF. Most of the articles were published before the release of the 2016 ESC HF guidelines,[12] and patients currently classified as having HFmrEF were included in the HFpEF category. The previous terminology with an EF cutoff of 50% is used here.

HFpEF can be diagnosed when a combination of clinical symptoms and signs, an EF more than 50%, and specific echocardiographic criteria are present. Echocardiography commonly shows either a structural heart disease (left atrial enlargement, left ventricular hypertrophy) or diastolic dysfunction, or both in patients with HFpEF.[12] Plasma galectin-3 levels tend to be similar in patients with HFpEF and HFrEF; however, studies show that galectin-3 values can directly relate to the severity of diastolic dysfunction[61] relate to what in patients with HFrEF?[58] A smaller study (N = 63 patients) also found a positive association between the serum galectin-3 levels and left ventricular diastolic filling properties, which was determined by late gadolinium-enhanced cardiac magnetic resonance imaging.[62] In the ALDOsterone Heart Failure (ALDO-DHF) study, increased galectin-3 plasma values directly correlated with cardiac function in patients with HFpEF. When galectin-3 level was more than 12.1 ng/mL at baseline, echocardiography revealed an enlarged left atrium and diastolic dysfunction (increased E/E′ ratio). However, there was no significant correlation of galectin-3 plasma values (N = 377) and spironolactone treatment in patients in the Aldo-DHF trial.[63] Because low values of NT-proBNP do not exclude HFpEF diagnosis, increased galectin-3 level can raise the suspicion of HFpEF and galectin-3 could therefore have a diagnostic utility in patients with HFpEF.[53,64]

Galectin-3 can also be used in prognosticating patients with HFpEF; galectin-3 was found to be the most accurate risk predictor of adverse events within 5 years in patients with HFpEF. A total of 1385 patients with HF were included in the study; 106 patients had a preserved ejection fraction.[65] These data support the results from the substudy of the COACH trial. The substudy (N initially 592, N = 114 with HFpEF), with a follow-up period of about 1.5 years, showed a higher predictive value of galectin-3 in HFpEF (EF>40%) for rehospitalization and death compared with HFrEF.[53]

GALECTIN-3 LEVELS IN SYSTEMIC DISORDERS

Although galectin-3 is used as a biomarker in HF, it seems to be neither a cardiac-specific biomarker nor a cardiac-specific protein. Variations of galectin-3 plasma levels depend on comorbidities, as shown in **Fig. 3**. Healthy individuals have the lowest baseline galectin-3 levels[25]; although galectin-3 levels increase in CHF[66] and ADHF,[34] the highest increases are observed in patients with end-stage kidney disease.[57] Increased galectin-3 levels are also observed in pulmonary conditions such as pneumonia and chronic obstructive pulmonary disease.[69,67] Very high galectin-3 levels are observed in sepsis.[68,69]

In otherwise healthy patients with HF, the FDA approved a plasma galectin-3 cutoff value of 17.8 ng/mL.[65] Correcting galectin-3 values for comorbidities/covariates or different circumstances is complex and clinicians have yet to understand the specific covariates. Although the predictive value of

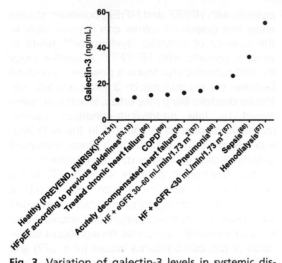

Fig. 3. Variation of galectin-3 levels in systemic diseases and in the general population. COPD, chronic obstructive pulmonary disease; eGFR, estimated glomerular filtration rate.

galectin-3 in patients with HF diminishes significantly after adjustment for renal function,[56] increased galectin-3 levels in patients with severe renal insufficiency independently predicted cardiovascular end points, infections, as well as all-cause mortality.[57] A minimal influence of diabetes mellitus on the predictive power of certain HF biomarkers, such as galectin-3, NT-proBNP, and hs-TNT, was found.[70] Diabetes was shown to influence the predictive value of ST2, because increased ST2 values were associated with an increased risk of HF in nondiabetic patients.[70]

RELATION BETWEEN SERUM GALECTIN-3 AND MYOCARDIAL GALECTIN-3 EXPRESSION

There are contradicting results concerning the direct relationship of plasma galectin-3 levels, myocardial galectin-3 expression, and myocardial fibrosis.

The relationship between plasma and myocardial galectin-3 values was evaluated in a canine model, which showed a direct relationship in a model of pressure overload.[61] An in vitro cell model also visualized an increase in galectin-3 level following stretch of cardiomyocytes,[61] suggesting that the heart can also be a source of this protein.

In a study involving 150 participants, a direct relationship between increased plasma galectin-3 (>14.6 ng/mL) and the amount of myocardial fibrosis could also be detected when imaging was done with contrast-enhanced cardiac MRI in patients with nonischemic dilated cardiomyopathy.[71]

Correlation of plasma and myocardial galectin-3 as a marker in nonischemic, noninflammatory

dilated cardiomyopathy (N = 40) versus inflammatory cardiomyopathy (N = 77) and its predictive capability in fibrosis was investigated recently. Galectin-3 levels in the plasma correlated neither with endomyocardial levels of galectin-3 nor with cardiac fibrosis in left ventricular biopsies of patients with the aforementioned types of cardiomyopathy. In the same patients, left ventricular biopsies revealed a direct correlation between myocardial galectin-3 expression and fibrosis.[72]

GALECTIN-3 AS A BIOTARGET

New research has highlighted the potential of modulating the development of cardiac fibrosis by blocking profibrotic proteins. Galectin-3 has been shown to be a specific modulator of different inflammatory and profibrotic processes in humans; clinical trials on galectin-3 inhibitors in different disease settings are currently ongoing, and these include several fibrotic disorders (eg, hepatic, renal, and pulmonary fibrosis) as well as malignancies (eg, colorectal cancer), as summarized in **Table 5**.

The upregulation of galectin-3 in rats prone to HF was shown to be strongly associated with decompensated HF.[17] Galectin-3 colocalized with macrophages, and upregulation of galectin-3 was the result of macrophage activation in heart tissue.[17] In another study, injecting galectin-3 into the pericardial sac of rats also triggered fibrosis and resulted in significant cardiac dysfunction.[73] Although usually associated with macrophages, a recent in vitro study also found galectin-3–expressing cultured cardiomyocytes after activation by protein kinase C.[74] Furthermore, galectin-3 knockout mice were resistant to angiotensin II–induced pressure overload and did not develop myocardial fibrosis and left ventricular dysfunction, compared with wild-type C57BL/6J mice, and this showed that galectin-3 was a culprit protein in cardiac fibrosis and HF.[75,76]

Different carbohydrate-based ligands of galectin-3, such as N-acetyllactosamine and modified citrus pectin (MCP), were studied in the setting of myocardial dysfunction. Treatment with N-acetyllactosamine, which binds to the CRD of galectin-3, decreased cardiac fibrosis, preserved the fractional shortening, reduced left ventricular end-diastolic pressure, reduced lung weight, and improved survival in HF-prone rats.[75] MCP, another galectin-3 inhibitor (as well as spironolactone), prevented cardiac dysfunction and hypertrophy, inhibited collagen type I synthesis, and decreased myocardial as well as renal collagen deposition in aldosterone-treated rats.[77] In addition, TD-139 a thiodigalactoside analogue, was studied in a phase IIa trial for the treatment

Table 5
Overview of galectin-3 inhibitors

Gal-3 Inhibitor	Mechanism of Action	Disease	Studies Trials
TD139	High-affinity inhibitor Binds to CBD Blocks TGF-β–induced β-catenin activation Diminishes lung fibrosis	Pulmonary fibrosis	Clinical phase II completed (NCT02257177)[67]
GR-MD-02	Proprietary galactoarabinorhamnogalacturonan polysaccharide polymer	Nonalcoholic steatosis hepatis/liver fibrosis	Murine model (higher potency than GM-CT-01 in treating liver fibrosis)[79]
	Binds to CBD		Clinical phase II[80] (NCT02421094)
	—	Psoriasis	Clinical phase II (NCT02407041)
	—	Metastatic melanoma Melanoma I	Clinical phase I (NCT02407041)
MCP /GCS 100	Polyvalent glycan inhibitor MCP-derived polysaccharide	NASH	IIb discontinued (La Jolla Pharmaceutical)
	Binds to CBD	Chronic kidney disease caused by diabetes	Clinical phase II (NCT02312050)
	Reversion of fibrosis, inhibition of cell migration, induction of apoptosis		
	—	Chronic lymphocytic leukemia[81]	Clinical phase II completed (NCT00514696)
	—	Diffuse large B-cell lymphoma[82]	Clinical phase I/II withdrawn (NCT00776802)
	—	Multiple myeloma[83]	Phase I (NCT00609817)
	—	Vascular fibrosis	Rat[84]
		Breast cancer	In vitro[85]
		Hypertension	Clinical study (NCT01960946)
		Prostate cancer	In vitro[85,86]
			Clinical phase III (recruiting) (NCT01681823)
		Osteoarthritis	Clinical phase III (NCT02800629)
		Ovarian cancer	In vitro[87]
		Renal cell carcinoma	In vitro[88]
		Chronic kidney disease	Clinical phase II (NCT02333955)
		Hypertension, acute kidney injury	In vitro[89]
		Liver metastasis of colon cancer	Mouse[90]

(continued on next page)

Table 5
(continued)

Gal-3 Inhibitor	Mechanism of Action	Disease	Studies Trials
N-acetyllactosamine	Attenuation of fibrosis	Cardiac fibrosis	Rat[75]
Lactulose L-leucine	Binds to CBD Inhibition of metastasis	Prostate cancer metastasis	Mouse[91]
Galectin-3C	Binds to CBD Inhibits tumor growth Reduces metastasis and tumor size	Multiple myeloma Breast cancer metastasis	Mouse[92] Mouse[93]
Td131_1	Binds to CBD Activation of apoptosis in tumor cells	Papillary thyroid cancer	In vitro[94]
N-acetyl-seryl-aspartyl-lysyl-proline (Ac-SDKP)	Prevention of cardiac fibrosis	Cardiac fibrosis	Rat[73]
Chemically modified, nonanticoagulant heparin derivatives	Binds to CBD Attenuation of galectin-3–mediated metastasis	Pulmonary metastasis of colon cancer and human melanoma	Mouse[95]
RN1	Binds to CBD	Pancreatic ductal adenocarcinoma	Mouse xenograft model[96]

Abbreviations: CBD, carbohydrate binding domain; MCP, modified citrus pectin; NASH, nonalcoholic steatohepatitis; TGF, transforming growth factor.
Adapted from de Boer RA, van der Velde AR, Mueller C, et al. Galectin-3: a modifiable risk factor in heart failure. Cardiovasc Drugs Ther 2014;28:243; with permission.

of idiopathic pulmonary fibrosis in the form of an inhaled powder (NCT02257177). Currently a phase IIb trial is being designed. Because this compound is not systemically available, its effects on (preventing) cardiac fibrosis have not been tested.

New systemically available galectin-3–specific inhibitors need to be developed and investigated. The possibilities are intriguing if a galectin-3 high affinity ? to what? and a preventive effect of HF as the only goal? were to be discovered. This breakthrough could be an opportunity to further reduce HF hospitalization, especially in patients with high galectin-3 levels, who, although treated with angiotensin II receptor blockers (valsartan),[49] did not show a reduced risk of hospitalization.

SUMMARY

In the last decades, galectin-3 has been intensely studied, and its role in various cellular and extracellular functions has been established. More recently, a role for galectin-3 in cardiac tissue remodeling has been explored. Specifically, galectin-3 plays a dominant role in cardiac inflammation, and fibrosis. Because galectin-3 is secreted into the systemic circulation, its levels can be measured, and its role as a biomarker was investigated in numerous studies in healthy subjects, in the elderly, and in patients with coronary artery disease, hypertension, renal disease, and predominantly HF. In a recent meta-analysis, galectin-3 was validated as a biomarker with independent prognostic value for mortality and HF rehospitalization. Currently clinicians lack tools acting on the increased risk conferred by galectin-3 (or any other biomarker), the clinical importance is minor. More promising, therefore in animal models, (genetic) deficiency of galectin-3 results in abolishment of tissue fibrosis, which was confirmed in numerous studies of renal, liver, lung, and cardiac fibrosis. Studies with oral inhibitors recapitulated this, and therefore the most promising outlook for galectin-3 is as an amenable target for tissue fibrosis. Several trials are underway with the aim of validating this concept; if proven useful, the authors predict it will have a major impact on the treatment of several multifactorial diseases.

ACKNOWLEDGMENTS

We would like to thank Peter Pozder for the language editing.

REFERENCES

1. Imran TF, Shin HJ, Mathenge N, et al. Meta-analysis of the usefulness of plasma galectin-3 to predict the risk of mortality in patients with heart failure and in the general population. Am J Cardiol 2017;119(1): 57–64.

2. De Boer RA, Voors AA, Muntendam P, et al. Galectin-3: a novel mediator of heart failure development and progression. Eur J Heart Fail 2009; 11(9):811–7.

3. de Boer RA, Yu L, van Veldhuisen DJ. Galectin-3 in cardiac remodeling and heart failure. Curr Heart Fail Rep 2010;7(1):1–8.

4. McCullough PA, Olobatoke A, Vanhecke TE. Galectin-3: a novel blood test for the evaluation and management of patients with heart failure. Rev Cardiovasc Med 2011;12(4):200–10.

5. De Boer RA, Edelmann F, Cohen-Solal A, et al. Galectin-3 in heart failure with preserved ejection fraction. Eur J Heart Fail 2013;15(10):1095–101.

6. Carrasco-Sánchez FJ, Páez-Rubio MI. Review of the prognostic value of galectin-3 in heart failure focusing on clinical utility of repeated testing. Mol Diagn Ther 2014;18(6):599–604.

7. Coburn E, Frishman W. Comprehensive review of the prognostic value of galectin-3 in heart failure. Cardiol Rev 2014;22(4):171–5.

8. Peacock WF, DiSomma S. Emergency department use of galectin-3. Crit Pathw Cardiol 2014;13(2): 73–7.

9. Mosterd A, Hoes AW. Clinical epidemiology of heart failure. Heart 2007;93(9):1137–46.

10. Screever EM, Meijers WC, van Veldhuisen DJ, et al. New developments in the pharmacotherapeutic management of heart failure in elderly patients: concerns and considerations. Expert Opin Pharmacother 2017;18(7):645–55.

11. Heidenreich PA, Albert NM, Allen LA, et al. Forecasting the impact of heart failure in the United States. Circ Heart Fail 2013;6(3):606–19.

12. Ponikowski P, Voors AA, Anker SD, et al. 2016 ESC guidelines for the diagnosis and treatment of acute and chronic heart failure. Eur Heart J 2016;37(27): 2129–200.

13. McMurray JJ, Adamopoulos S, Anker SD, et al. ESC guidelines for the diagnosis and treatment of acute and chronic heart failure 2012: the Task Force for the Diagnosis and Treatment of Acute and Chronic Heart Failure 2012 of the European Society of Cardiology. Developed in collaboration with the Heart Failure Association (HFA) of the ESC. Eur Heart J 2012; 33(14):1787–847.

14. Suthahar N, Meijers WC, Silljé HHW, et al. From inflammation to fibrosis — molecular and cellular mechanisms of myocardial tissue remodelling and perspectives on differential treatment opportunities. Curr Heart Fail Rep 2017;14(4):235–50.

15. Huis In 't Veld AE, de Man FS, van Rossum AC, et al. How to diagnose heart failure with preserved ejection fraction: the value of invasive stress testing. Neth Heart J 2016;24(4):244–51.

16. Yancy CW, Jessup M, Bozkurt B, et al. 2013 ACCF/AHA guideline for the management of heart failure: a report of the American College of Cardiology Foundation/American Heart Association Task Force on Practice Guidelines. Circulation 2013;128(16): e240–327.

17. Sharma UC, Pokharel S, van Brakel TJ, et al. Galectin-3 marks activated macrophages in failure-prone hypertrophied hearts and contributes to cardiac dysfunction. Circulation 2004;110(19):3121–8.

18. Meijers WC, van der Velde AR, de Boer RA. The ARCHITECT galectin-3 assay: comparison with other automated and manual assays for the measurement of circulating galectin-3 levels in heart failure. Expert Rev Mol Diagn 2014;14(3):257–66.

19. Christenson RH, Duh SH, Wu AH, et al. Multi-center determination of galectin-3 assay performance characteristics: anatomy of a novel assay for use in heart failure. Clin Biochem 2010;43(7–8):683–90.

20. BGM Galectin-3® Test. Available at: http://www.bg-medicine.com/bgm-galectin-3-test. Accessed September 24, 2017.

21. R&D Systems®. Quantikine ® ELISA. Available at: https://resources.rndsystems.com/pdfs/datasheets/dgal30.pdf. Accessed September 24, 2017.

22. La'ulu SL, Apple FS, Murakami MM, et al. Performance characteristics of the ARCHITECT galectin-3 assay. Clin Biochem 2013;46(1–2):119–22.

23. Gaze DC, Prante C, Dreier J, et al. Analytical evaluation of the automated galectin-3 assay on the Abbott ARCHITECT immunoassay instruments. Clin Chem Lab Med 2014;52(6):919–26.

24. Gruson D, Mancini M, Ahn SA, et al. Galectin-3 testing: validity of a novel automated assay in heart failure patients with reduced ejection fraction. Clin Chim Acta 2014;429:189–93.

25. Meijers WC, van der Velde AR, Muller Kobold AC, et al. Variability of biomarkers in patients with chronic heart failure and healthy controls. Eur J Heart Fail 2017;19(3):357–65.

26. Schindler EI, Szymanski JJ, Hock KG, et al. Short- and long-term biologic variability of galectin-3 and other cardiac biomarkers in patients with stable heart failure and healthy adults. Clin Chem 2016; 62(2):360–6.

27. de Boer RA, van Veldhuisen DJ, Gansevoort RT, et al. The fibrosis marker galectin-3 and outcome in the general population. J Intern Med 2012; 272(1):55–64.

28. McEvoy JW, Chen Y, Halushka MK, et al. Galectin-3 and risk of heart failure and death in blacks and whites. J Am Heart Assoc 2016;5(5).

29. Ho JE, Liu C, Lyass A, et al. Galectin-3, a marker of cardiac fibrosis, predicts incident heart failure in the community. J Am Coll Cardiol 2012;60(14):1249–56.

30. Daniels LB, Clopton P, Laughlin GA, et al. Galectin-3 is independently associated with cardiovascular mortality in community-dwelling older adults without known cardiovascular disease: the Rancho Bernardo Study. Am Heart J 2014;167(5):674–82.e1.

31. Jagodzinski A, Havulinna AS, Appelbaum S, et al. Predictive value of galectin-3 for incident cardiovascular disease and heart failure in the population-based FINRISK 1997 cohort. Int J Cardiol 2015; 192:33–9.

32. van der Velde AR, Meijers WC, Ho JE, et al. Serial galectin-3 and future cardiovascular disease in the general population. Heart 2016;102(14): 1134–41.

33. Maggioni AP, Dahlström U, Filippatos G, et al. EURObservational Research Programme: regional differences and 1-year follow-up results of the Heart Failure Pilot Survey (ESC-HF Pilot). Eur J Heart Fail 2013;15(7):808–17.

34. Shah RV, Chen-Tournoux AA, Picard MH, et al. Galectin-3, cardiac structure and function, and long-term mortality in patients with acutely decompensated heart failure. Eur J Heart Fail 2010;12(8):826–32.

35. Mueller T, Gegenhuber A, Leitner I, et al. Diagnostic and prognostic accuracy of galectin-3 and soluble ST2 for acute heart failure. Clin Chim Acta 2016; 463:158–64.

36. Meijers WC, de Boer RA, van Veldhuisen DJ, et al. Biomarkers and low risk in heart failure. Data from COACH and TRIUMPH. Eur J Heart Fail 2015; 17(2):1271–82.

37. van Kimmenade RR, Januzzi JL Jr, Ellinor PT, et al. Utility of amino-terminal pro-brain natriuretic peptide, galectin-3, and apelin for the evaluation of patients with acute heart failure. J Am Coll Cardiol 2006;48(6):1217–24.

38. Eurlings LW, Sanders-van Wijk S, van Kimmenade R, et al. Multimarker strategy for short-term risk assessment in patients with dyspnea in the emergency department: the MARKED (Multi mARKer Emergency Dyspnea)-risk score. J Am Coll Cardiol 2012;60(17):1668–77.

39. Fermann GJ, Lindsell CJ, Storrow AB, et al. Galectin 3 complements BNP in risk stratification in acute heart failure. Biomarkers 2012;17(8):706–13.

40. De Berardinis B, Magrini L, Zampini G, et al. Usefulness of combining galectin-3 and BIVA assessments in predicting short- and long-term events in patients admitted for acute heart failure. Biomed Res Int 2014;2014:983098.

41. Carrasco-Sánchez FJ, Aramburu-Bodas O, Salamanca-Bautista P, et al. Predictive value of serum galectin-3 levels in patients with acute heart failure with preserved ejection fraction. Int J Cardiol 2013; 169(3):177–82.

42. Sudharshan S, Novak E, Hock K, et al. Use of biomarkers to predict readmission for congestive heart failure. Am J Cardiol 2017;119(3):445–51.

43. Miró Ò, González de la Presa B, Herrero-Puente P, et al. The GALA study: relationship between galectin-3 serum levels and short- and long-term outcomes of patients with acute heart failure. Biomarkers 2017;5804:1–9.

44. Meijers WC, Januzzi JL, Defilippi C, et al. Elevated plasma galectin-3 is associated with near-term rehospitalization in heart failure: a pooled analysis of 3 clinical trials. Am Heart J 2014;167(6):853–60.e4.

45. Demissei BG, Cotter G, Prescott MF, et al. A multimarker multi-time point-based risk stratification strategy in acute heart failure: results from the RELAX-AHF trial. Eur J Heart Fail 2017; 19(8):1001–10.

46. Demissei BG, Valente MA, Cleland JG, et al. Optimizing clinical use of biomarkers in high-risk acute heart failure patients. Eur J Heart Fail 2016;18(3): 269–80.

47. Adams PE, Martinez ME, Vickerie JL, et al. Summary Health Statistics for the U. S. Population: National Health Interview Survey. Vital Health Stat 10 2011;(251):1–117.

48. Gullestad L, Ueland T, Kjekshus J, et al. Galectin-3 predicts response to statin therapy in the Controlled Rosuvastatin Multinational Trial in Heart Failure (CORONA). Eur Heart J 2012;33(18):2290–6.

49. Anand IS, Rector TS, Kuskowski M, et al. Baseline and serial measurements of galectin-3 in patients with heart failure: relationship to prognosis and effect of treatment with valsartan in the Val-HeFT. Eur J Heart Fail 2013;15(5):511–8.

50. Lin YH, Lin LY, Wu YW, et al. The relationship between serum galectin-3 and serum markers of cardiac extracellular matrix turnover in heart failure patients. Clin Chim Acta 2009;409(1–2): 96–9.

51. Lok DJ, Van Der Meer P, de la Porte PW, et al. Prognostic value of galectin-3, a novel marker of fibrosis, in patients with chronic heart failure: data from the DEAL-HF study. Clin Res Cardiol 2010; 99(5):323–8.

52. Van Der Velde AR, Gullestad L, Ueland T, et al. Prognostic value of changes in galectin-3 levels over time in patients with heart failure data from CORONA and COACH. Circ Heart Fail 2013;6(2):219–26.

53. de Boer RA, Lok DJ, Jaarsma T, et al. Predictive value of plasma galectin-3 levels in heart failure with reduced and preserved ejection fraction. Ann Med 2011;43(1):60–8.

54. Miller WL, Saenger AK, Grill DE, et al. Prognostic value of serial measurements of soluble suppression of tumorigenicity 2 and galectin-3 in ambulatory patients with chronic heart failure. J Card Fail 2016; 22(4):249–55.

55. Billebeau G, Vodovar N, Sadoune M, et al. Effects of a cardiac rehabilitation programme on plasma cardiac biomarkers in patients with chronic heart failure. Eur J Prev Cardiol 2017;24(11):1127–35.

56. Zamora E, Lupón J, de Antonio M, et al. Renal function largely influences galectin-3 prognostic value in heart failure. Int J Cardiol 2014;177(1):171–7.

57. Drechsler C, Delgado G, Wanner C, et al. Galectin-3, renal function, and clinical outcomes: results from the LURIC and 4D studies. J Am Soc Nephrol 2015;26(9):2213–21.

58. Stoltze Gaborit F, Bosselmann H, Kistorp C, et al. Galectin 3: association to neurohumoral activity, echocardiographic parameters and renal function in outpatients with heart failure. BMC Cardiovasc Disord 2016;16:117.

59. Ahmad T, Fiuzat M, Neely B, et al. Biomarkers of myocardial stress and fibrosis as predictors of mode of death in patients with chronic heart failure. JACC Heart Fail 2014;2(3):260–8.

60. Bayes-Genis A, de Antonio M, Vila J, et al. Head-to-head comparison of 2 myocardial fibrosis biomarkers for long-term heart failure risk stratification: ST2 versus galectin-3. J Am Coll Cardiol 2014;63(2):158–66.

61. Wu CK, Su MY, Lee JK, et al. Galectin-3 level and the severity of cardiac diastolic dysfunction using cellular and animal models and clinical indices. Sci Rep 2015;5:17007.

62. Lepojärvi ES, Piira OP, Pääkkö E, et al. Serum PINP, PIIINP, galectin-3, and ST2 as surrogates of myocardial fibrosis and echocardiographic left ventricular diastolic filling properties. Front Physiol 2015;6:200.

63. Edelmann F, Holzendorf V, Wachter R, et al. Galectin-3 in patients with heart failure with preserved ejection fraction: results from the Aldosterone Receptor Blockade in Diastolic Heart Failure (Aldo-DHF) trial. Eur J Heart Fail 2015;17(2):214–23 (Ci).

64. Meijers WC, van der Velde AR, de Boer RA. Biomarkers in heart failure with preserved ejection fraction. Neth Heart J 2016;24(4):252–8.

65. French B, Wang L, Ky B, et al. Prognostic value of galectin-3 for adverse outcomes in chronic heart failure. J Card Fail 2016;22(4):256–62.

66. Boulogne M, Sadoune M, Launay JM, et al. Inflammation versus mechanical stretch biomarkers over time in acutely decompensated heart failure with reduced ejection fraction. Int J Cardiol 2017;226: 53–9.

67. Meyer KC. Pulmonary fibrosis, part II: state-of-the-art patient management. Expert Rev Respir Med 2017;11(5):361–76.

68. Mueller T, Leitner I, Egger M, et al. Association of the biomarkers soluble ST2, galectin-3 and growth-differentiation factor-15 with heart failure and other non-cardiac diseases. Clin Chim Acta 2015;445: 155–60.

69. Agoston-Coldea L, Lupu S, Petrovai D, et al. Correlations between echocardiographic parameters of right ventricular dysfunction and galectin-3 in

patients with chronic obstructive pulmonary disease and pulmonary hypertension. Med Ultrason 2015;17(4):487–95.

70. Alonso N, Lupón J, Barallat J, et al. Impact of diabetes on the predictive value of heart failure biomarkers. Cardiovasc Diabetol 2016;15(1):151.

71. Vergaro G, Del Franco A, Giannoni A, et al. Galectin-3 and myocardial fibrosis in nonischemic dilated cardiomyopathy. Int J Cardiol 2015;184(1):96–100.

72. Besler C, Lang D, Urban D, et al. Plasma and cardiac galectin-3 in patients with heart failure reflects both inflammation and fibrosis: implications for its use as a biomarker. Circ Heart Fail 2017;10(3).

73. Liu YH, D'Ambrosio M, Liao TD, et al. N-acetyl-seryl-aspartyl-lysyl-proline prevents cardiac remodeling and dysfunction induced by galectin-3, a mammalian adhesion/growth-regulatory lectin. Am J Physiol Heart Circ Physiol 2009;296:H404–12.

74. Song X, Qian X, Shen M, et al. Protein kinase C promotes cardiac fibrosis and heart failure by modulating galectin-3 expression. Biochim Biophys Acta 2015;1853(2):513–21.

75. Yu L, Ruifrok WP, Meissner M, et al. Genetic and pharmacological inhibition of galectin-3 prevents cardiac remodeling by interfering with myocardial fibrogenesis. Circ Heart Fail 2013;6(1):107–17.

76. González GE, Rhaleb NE, D'Ambrosio MA, et al. Cardiac-deleterious role of galectin-3 in chronic angiotensin II-induced hypertension. Am J Physiol Heart Circ Physiol 2016;311(5):H1287–96.

77. Calvier L, Martinez-Martinez E, Miana M, et al. The impact of galectin-3 inhibition on aldosterone-induced cardiac and renal injuries. JACC Heart Fail 2015;3(1):59–67.

78. van der Velde AR, Meijers WC, van den Heuvel ER, et al. Determinants of temporal changes in galectin-3 level in the general population: Data of PREVEND. Int J Cardiol 2016;222:385–90.

79. Traber PG, Zomer E. Therapy of experimental NASH and fibrosis with galectin inhibitors. PLoS One 2013;8(12):e83481.

80. Rotman Y, Sanyal AJ. Current and upcoming pharmacotherapy for non-alcoholic fatty liver disease. Gut 2017;66(1):180–90.

81. Cotter F, Smith DA, Boyd TE, et al. Single-agent activity of GCS-100, a first-in-class galectin-3 antagonist, in elderly patients with relapsed chronic lymphocytic leukemia. J Clin Oncol 2009;27(15_suppl):7006.

82. Clark MC, Pang M, Hsu DK, et al. Galectin-3 binds to CD45 on diffuse large B-cell lymphoma cells to regulate susceptibility to cell death. Blood 2012;120(23):4635–44.

83. Chauhan D, Li G, Podar K, et al. A novel carbohydrate-based therapeutic GCS-100 overcomes bortezomib resistance and enhances dexamethasone-induced apoptosis in multiple myeloma cells. Cancer Res 2005;65(18):8350–8.

84. Calvier L, Miana M, Reboul P, et al. Galectin-3 mediates aldosterone-induced vascular fibrosis. Arterioscler Thromb Vasc Biol 2013;33(1):67–75.

85. Jiang J, Eliaz I, Sliva D. Synergistic and additive effects of modified citrus pectin with two polybotanical compounds, in the suppression of invasive behavior of human breast and prostate cancer cells. Integr Cancer Ther 2013;12(2):145–52.

86. Wang Y, Nangia-Makker P, Balan V, et al. Calpain activation through galectin-3 inhibition sensitizes prostate cancer cells to cisplatin treatment. Cell Death Dis 2010;1:e101.

87. Hossein G, Keshavarz M, Ahmadi S, et al. Synergistic effects of PectaSol-C modified citrus pectin an inhibitor of galectin-3 and paclitaxel on apoptosis of human SKOV-3 ovarian cancer cells. Asian Pac J Cancer Prev 2013;14(12):7561–8.

88. Xu ZZ, Wang M, Wang YJ, et al. Effect of nitrotyrosine on renal expressions of NF-kappaB, MCP-1 and TGF-beta1 in rats with diabetic nephropathy. Nan Fang Yi Ke Da Xue Bao 2013;33(3):346–50.

89. Kolatsi-Joannou M, Price KL, Winyard PJ, et al. Modified citrus pectin reduces galectin-3 expression and disease severity in experimental acute kidney injury. PLoS One 2011;6(4):e18683.

90. Liu HY, Huang ZL, Yang GH, et al. Inhibitory effect of modified citrus pectin on liver metastases in a mouse colon cancer model. World J Gastroenterol 2008;14(48):7386–91.

91. Glinskii OV, Sud S, Mossine VV, et al. Inhibition of prostate cancer bone metastasis by synthetic TF antigen mimic/galectin-3 inhibitor lactulose-L-leucine. Neoplasia 2012;14(1):65–73.

92. Mirandola L, Yu Y, Chui K, et al. Galectin-3C inhibits tumor growth and increases the anticancer activity of bortezomib in a murine model of human multiple myeloma. PLoS One 2011;6(7):e21811.

93. John CM, Leffler H, Kahl-Knutsson B, et al. Truncated galectin-3 inhibits tumor growth and metastasis in orthotopic nude mouse model of human breast cancer. Clin Cancer Res 2003;9(6):2374–83.

94. Lin CI, Whang EE, Donner DB, et al. Galectin-3 targeted therapy with a small molecule inhibitor activates apoptosis and enhances both chemosensitivity and radiosensitivity in papillary thyroid cancer. Mol Cancer Res 2009;7(10):1655–62.

95. Duckworth CA, Guimond SE, Sindrewicz P, et al. Chemically modified, non-anticoagulant heparin derivatives are potent galectin-3 binding inhibitors and inhibit circulating galectin-3-promoted metastasis. Oncotarget 2015;6(27):23671–87.

96. Zhang L, Wang P, Qin Y, et al. RN1, a novel galectin-3 inhibitor, inhibits pancreatic cancer cell growth in vitro and in vivo via blocking galectin-3 associated signaling pathways. Oncogene 2017;36(9):1297–308.

Proteomic Biomarkers of Heart Failure

Muhammad Zubair Israr, MSc[a,1], Liam M. Heaney, PhD[a,1], Toru Suzuki, MD, PhD[a,b],*

KEYWORDS

- Biomarkers • Heart failure • Prognosis • Diagnosis • Proteomics

KEY POINTS

- Heart failure is associated with significant morbidity and mortality.
- Biomarkers are commonly used for diagnostic and prognostic purposes.
- Protein-based biomarkers have been identified to aid clinicians in the early diagnosis of heart failure and provide added information for prognosis.
- Proteomics is an ever-expanding field that uses techniques to measure a wide range of proteins and peptides in the search to identify potential protein biomarkers.

INTRODUCTION

It is estimated that in excess of 20,000 protein-coding genes are responsible for the presence of more than 1 million proteins found in biological matrices.[1] The measurement of these proteins, commonly in plasma, serum, urine, saliva, and tissue samples,[2] has provided critical advancements in medical science through the development of diagnostic and prognostic assays for patients presenting with, or at risk of, a multitude of diseases.[3] The use of protein measurements has been particularly beneficial for the assessment of cardiovascular disease, with the notable inclusion of natriuretic peptides and troponin isoforms in clinical decision making for heart failure (HF)[4] and acute coronary syndromes (ACS),[5] respectively. Clinical measurements of endogenous biological substances, such as proteins, lipids, and metabolites, are commonly referred to as biomarkers and provide pathophysiologic information through an associative or direct mechanistic interaction with the diseased system, organ, or tissue.[6] The relationships of protein biomarkers with disease allow physicians to assess the presence, severity, and/or prognosis of a condition with improved precision and accuracy.[7]

The progression in medical diagnosis and treatment of HF has been heavily influenced by the inclusion of protein biomarker analyses, with measurement of natriuretic peptides commonly used in hospitals worldwide.[8] HF is a major worldwide epidemic associated with high morbidity, mortality, and health care costs affecting more than 23 million people, especially those aged 65 years or older[9]; therefore, any improvements in diagnosis, prognosis, and therapeutic monitoring using protein measurements provide direct improvements in patient care and outcome, as well as economic burden. Difficulties in HF diagnoses exist because of the multifactorial pathophysiology (eg, cardiac stress and injury, neurohormonal activation, and endothelial congestion), and because the signs and symptoms may not arise during early stages of the disease.[10,11] Current guidelines suggest that patients presenting with suspected HF should

Disclosure: The authors have no disclosures.

[a] Department of Cardiovascular Sciences, NIHR Biomedical Research Centre, University of Leicester, Glenfield Hospital, Groby Road, Leicester LE3 9QP, UK; [b] Jichi Medical University, 3311-1 Yakushiji, Shimotsuke-shi, Tochigi-ken 329-0498, Japan

[1] M.Z. Israr and L.M. Heaney contributed equally to this article.

* Corresponding author. Department of Cardiovascular Sciences, NIHR Leicester Biomedical Research Centre, University of Leicester, Glenfield Hospital, Leicester LE3 9QP, UK.

E-mail address: ts263@le.ac.uk

heartfailure.theclinics.com

be referred for measurement of circulating natriuretic peptides to aid in diagnosis of the condition.[12]

The development and pathophysiology of HF is associated with changes in the expressions of an array of metabolic, signaling, and structural proteins.[13] Although there are several protein-based assays currently used in clinical laboratories, extensive research is being performed to isolate and identify novel protein biomarkers associated with HF in a bid to improve sensitivity and/or specificity of biomarker information. Leading these discovery-led investigations are mass spectrometry (MS)–based assays, which involve a nontargeted approach to protein measurement and come under the remit of proteomics. These assays measure all detectable proteins that are expressed by a cell, tissue, or organism, known as the proteome, and reflect levels present at the time of sample collection.[14,15]

PROTEOMIC BIOMARKER DISCOVERY

For discovery-led proteomics investigations, the initial phase involves methods using either a widespan-targeted or nontargeted approach in order to measure a large number of proteins and/or peptides from various biological sample types. This method generates a list of numerous proteins that are identified as associated with the condition being investigated and, therefore, are selected as candidate proteins for subsequent verification experiments. Although many candidate protein biomarkers may be identified through these experimental workflows, very few survive the rigorous validation processes leading to the development of high-throughput assays for measurement.[16] MS is the most widely used instrumentation for nontargeted discovery and identification of potential protein biomarkers. It allows quantitative and qualitative analysis, and peptide sequencing and identification, with great accuracy and sensitivity.[17] Proteomic workflows vary greatly across investigations, including sample preparation, chromatographic gradients, and inclusion of complementary analytical techniques such as ion mobility spectrometry. Furthermore, differences across studies in data processing and statistical testing can lead to misidentification or masking of candidate biomarkers. These widely varied approaches provide limitations in that biomarker identification may not be reproducible across multiple methods, complicating the validation process for novel protein biomarkers. Typically, MS method workflows include fractionation to crudely separate proteins in the sample, removal of highly abundant proteins such as albumin in plasma

samples, further separation of each fraction using liquid chromatography, and MS using electrospray ionization (ESI) in positive ion mode coupled to accurate mass analyzers such as time of flight (ToF) and orbitrap.[18] Alternatively, gel-based approaches are initially used to separate proteins by their isoelectric points and then by mass using polyacrylamide gel (sodium dodecyl sulfate polyacrylamide gel electrophoresis [SDS-PAGE]), followed by staining, excising, digesting using trypsin, and analysis by MS.[19] Following identification of candidate biomarkers, mass spectral data are cross-referenced with large-scale databases to confirm protein identification. Errors in protein quantitation in global discovery techniques can be associated throughout the analytical work flow from sample preparation to analysis. To assist in reducing these errors, isotopic labeling of internal protein standards can allow the relative quantitation of multiple proteins. Examples of these include metabolic labeling (^{15}N) and isotope-coded affinity tags; however, they lack accuracy and precision and more reliable approaches for sample-wide quantitation are required.[20]

Traditional nontargeted MS–based methods are important in candidate biomarker identification; however, complex sample preparation and analysis steps create a time-consuming process that limits the throughput required for larger-scale validation studies. Once a list of candidate biomarkers is produced, a shift toward targeted MS approaches allows improved specificity, reproducibility, and quantitation of candidates, and also drastically reduces the analytical run time. A commonly used approach for targeted MS is to develop assays using selective reaction monitoring (SRM) or multiple reaction monitoring (MRM), in which a single ion (SRM) or up to 5 fragment ions (MRM) are monitored in association with a specific product ion, typically using a triple quadrupole MS system, which is able to provide enhanced discriminating power, leading to increased sensitivity, absolute quantitation,[21,22] and improved cross-compatibility between instrumentation.[23] Aside from ESI-MS, matrix-assisted laser desorption ionization (MALDI) ToF–based MS is used for targeted MS, in which proteins of interest can be isolated using immunoprecipitation or liquid chromatography before spotting onto a target plate for analysis. Several targeted protein analyses using MALDI have been reported,[24,25] including an application in clinical studies.[26,27] Before commercialization, targeted protein experiments must replicate the results observed from the nontargeted investigations, as well as expanding to larger sample cohorts including diseased and nondiseased populations to validate as a biomarker of a condition and to understand normal ranges and potential disease cutoff values.

Because protein expressions show multifaceted temporospatial characteristics driven by responses to physical and/or biological stimuli, there are several complexities involved in the process of identifying a novel protein biomarker. In order to confirm the utility of a candidate biomarker for a clinical purpose, several steps must be achieved, including discovery, qualification, verification, optimization, and validation, followed by commercialization and distribution of assays[28] (**Fig. 1**). Although the discovery of novel proteins is driven by mass spectrometric methods, validation and commercialization more frequently involve traditional antibody-based techniques such as enzyme-linked immunosorbent assay (ELISA), Western blotting, and immunoblotting, with the less common use of MS-based methods in a clinical setting dictated by obstacles in regulatory approval and cross-site/cross-equipment reproducibility.[29] Regardless of the most suitable analytical method, a successful biomarker must be easily measured, low cost, patient friendly, and show high levels of sensitivity and specificity for its purpose (eg, diagnosis, prognosis).[30]

This article highlights the current clinical uses of protein biomarkers in HF (**Fig. 2**) and discusses the application of targeted and nontargeted proteomic investigations to discover and develop novel biomarkers centered on using a personalized medicine approach for improved prognostic information.

MARKERS OF CARDIAC STRESS
B-Type Natriuretic Peptide/N-Terminal Pro–B-Type Natriuretic Peptide

B-type natriuretic peptide (BNP) is perhaps the most widely used biomarker for cardiac stress. It is a central component in cardiovascular homeostasis and is released from the cardiomyocytes, primarily located in the ventricles, in response to stress and stretch of the cardiac muscle.[31] After binding to specific receptors, BNP is activated and drives a reduction in systemic vascular resistance, antagonizes the actions of the renin-angiotensin-aldosterone system, and promotes vasodilation and natriuresis.[32] BNP has been studied extensively for its role as a diagnostic[33–35] and prognostic[36–38] biomarker in HF, including both chronic patients and acute decompensated admissions. However, an important limitation of BNP for HF diagnosis is that circulating levels may become increased in response to alternative disorders such as renal dysfunction, left ventricular hypertrophy, and right ventricular dysfunction.[39] Furthermore, because factors such as sex, age, and body mass index are also associated with fluctuations in BNP levels, accurate interpretation of circulating concentrations is crucial.[40]

In addition to uses in diagnosis and prognosis, BNP has shown utility for the monitoring of patients treated with diuretics and vasodilators such as angiotensin-converting enzyme inhibitors,[41] angiotensin-II receptor antagonists,[42] and aldosterone inhibitors.[43] Circulating BNP levels

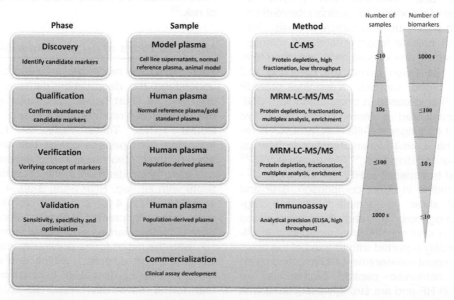

Fig. 1. Protein biomarker discovery pipeline of novel candidate biomarkers. ELISA, enzyme-linked immune-sorbent assay; LC-MS/MS, liquid chromatography tandem mass spectrometry.

MARKERS OF NEUROHORMONAL ACTIVATION:

- Copeptin
- Matrix metalloprotease

MARKERS OF REMODELLING:

- Galectin-3
- GDF-15

MARKERS OF INFLAMMATION OR INJURY:

- Troponin (T and I)
- H-FABP
- CRP
- TNF-α
- IL-6

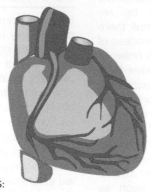

MARKERS OF ASSOCIATED COMORBIDITIES:

RENAL MARKERS:

- Cystatin C
- NGAL
- PENK

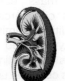

MARKERS OF CARDIAC STRESS:

- BNP/NTproBNP
- Molecular forms of BNP
- ANP
- ST2
- MRproADM

PULMONARY MARKER:

- Procalcitonin

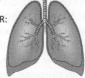

Fig. 2. Protein biomarkers of heart failure and their various pathophysiologic associations. ANP, atrial natriuretic peptide; BNP, B-type natriuretic peptide; CRP, C-reactive protein; GDF-15, growth differentiation factor-15; H-FABP, heart-type fatty acid–binding protein; IL-6, interleukin-6; MRproADM, midregional proadrenomedullin; NGAL, neutrophil gelatinase-associated lipocalin; NTproBNP, N-terminal pro–B-type natriuretic peptide; PENK, proenkephalin; TNF-α, tumor necrosis factor-α.

are known to decrease rapidly following successful treatment strategies, therefore repeat measurements of BNP concentrations provide an observation of responses to medical interventions.

Although widely used in clinical analysis, BNP has a short half-life (approximately 20 minutes) when present in the circulation[44] and, therefore, care must be taken during the sampling and storing of blood samples. N-terminal proBNP (NTproBNP) is released in conjunction with BNP and is considered a more stable alternative because of its longer half-life.[45] NTproBNP is reported to have similar characteristics to BNP as a biomarker for diagnosis,[46–48] prognosis,[42,46,49] and guided treatment[50] in HF.

When studied in direct comparison, BNP and NTproBNP show comparable utility for diagnosis,[42] prognosis,[51,52] and biomarker-guided therapy[53] in chronic HF, with reductions in all-cause mortality reported with titration of therapies based on repeat measurements. Circulating levels of these natriuretic peptide biomarkers are increased in HF and are strongly associated with disease severity and myocardial stretch.[54] Studies, such as the Valsartan Heart Failure Trial

(Val-HeFT), have also shown BNP and NTproBNP to provide superior prognostic information compared with alternative neurohormonal markers of risk.[55]

Molecular Forms of B-Type Natriuretic Peptide

There have been recent research efforts to further understand the degradation pathways of BNP and, with its short half-life in circulation, experiments have also reported the presence of its molecular forms. These molecular forms are truncated BNP peptide chains that are synthesized by the proteolysis of end-chain amino acids and have been identified in the circulation of patients with HF (eg, BNP 3-29, 3-30, 4-29, 5-29), with BNP 3-32, 4-32 and 5-32 reported as the most commonly present.[56] These molecular forms have recently emerged as potential biomarkers for HF, with the major forms previously implicated in ischemic heart disease,[57] which is a major risk factor for development of HF. Furthermore, molecular forms have been reported to associate more closely with clinically measured BNP levels compared with the parent BNP molecule

(BNP 1-32). This finding suggests that the specificity of clinical BNP assays is not unique to BNP 1-32, and that the combination of intact and molecular forms of BNP is a more accurate representation of circulating BNP measurements.[58] More recently, molecular forms of BNP have shown prognostic qualities superior to or comparable with NTproBNP for risk stratification of patients with acute HF. BNP 3-32, 4-32, and notably 5-32 were able to independently predict adverse outcome of patients at 6 months and 1 year, outlining its use as a biomarker to guide outpatient management.[27] However, direct mechanistic actions of these truncated forms, along with the dynamics and kinetics of their degradation pathways, are not currently understood and remain areas of current research.

Atrial Natriuretic Peptide

Atrial natriuretic peptide (ANP) is primarily secreted from the atria and has similar physiological properties to BNP. It is thought to play a role in early HF by preserving the compensated state of left ventricular dysfunction.[59] Although reported to be a prognostic indicator in HF, studies have reported ANP as inferior to BNP primarily because of its decreased stability in circulation and its insensitivity to levels of HF severity.[60,61] Other forms of ANP, such as N-terminal ANP, N-terminal pro-ANP, and midregional pro-ANP (MRproANP), have also been shown to suggest diagnostic and prognostic roles in HF.[61-63] MRproANP has far greater stability in circulation and therefore could prove more suitable for use as a biomarker compared with ANP. An investigation using The Biomarkers in Acute Heart Failure (BACH) cohort reported that MRproANP was a suitable diagnostic and prognostic biomarker in dyspneic patients, with results comparable with those of BNP.[63] Furthermore, additional studies have also indicated that MRproANP provides additive prognostic information to NTproBNP in chronic HF[64] and as a diagnostic marker of acute destabilized HF in patients with dyspnea, again reporting comparable results with the use of both BNP and NTproBNP.[65]

ST2

ST2 is a member of the interleukin (IL)-1 receptor family and has been identified as the target for IL-33, which is expressed under biochemical stress of the heart.[66] ST2 is basally expressed by cardiomyocytes and is detectable in circulation in its soluble form, levels of which are increased in response to mechanical stress of the heart.[67] Its utility has been recognized in HF as an independent predictor of mortality or need for transplant in patients with severe chronic HF (New York Heart Association [NYHA] class III/ IV),[67] as well as providing prognostic information for patients with acute HF when combined with natriuretic peptides,[68] suggesting applicability as a biomarker in combination with current clinical testing strategies (eg, BNP and NTproBNP). Furthermore, although NTproBNP showed improved diagnostic accuracy for patients with acute HF, the PRIDE (Pro-Brain Natriuretic Peptide Investigation of Dyspnea in the Emergency Department) study showed that ST2 was a suitable biomarker to predict 1-year mortality in dyspneic patients, irrespective of a positive or negative diagnosis of acute destabilizing HF,[69] suggesting a more generalized biomarker function that can be further refined when applying a multi-biomarker approach.

Midregional Proadrenomedullin

Adrenomedullin (ADM) is a peptide hormone that has natriuretic, vasodilatory, and hypotensive effects on the heart, with plasma concentrations increased in response to these effects, such as in chronic HF.[70] However, because ADM is unstable in circulation, its midregional prohormone fragment midregional proadrenomedullin (MRproADM) is often measured to perform an indirect quantitation.[71] It has reported a varied role in prognosis, providing information for short-term (30 days) and long-term (4 years) prognosis but less success for midrange predictions of outcome (1 year).[72] MRproADM has also been successfully shown as a prognostic biomarker for patients with acute HF presenting with dyspnea.[73] In this study it was reported as a superior biomarker to both BNP and NTproBNP for the short-term prediction of mortality (90 days) as well as for subsequent patient rehospitalization.[73] Data suggest that it has a suitable role for use in HF prognosis; however, further investigations to confirm its superiority to current biomarkers are warranted.

MARKERS OF INFLAMMATION OR INJURY
Troponin

Troponin proteins are found in cardiac and skeletal muscle tissue and are involved in the regulation of actin and myosin interactions during muscle contraction. Cardiac troponin I (cTnI) and cardiac troponin T (cTnT) have unique isoforms that exist only in cardiac muscle, allowing the measurement of these specific isoforms to provide information in cardiovascular disease, notably as diagnostic biomarkers for ACS.[74] However, development of high-sensitivity troponin assays have further allowed the measurement of increased cTnI/cTnT levels in patients with HF,[75,76] with increased concentrations associated with poor outcome. High-sensitivity assays for cTnT have been applied for prognosis in chronic HF, with circulating concentrations able to predict mortality and hospitalization in stabilized patients.[77] Furthermore, cTnT has been shown as a suitable marker to reflect myocardial damage in severe chronic HF,[78] to risk stratify patients on admission for subsequent mortality and morbidity,[79] and to identify patients at high risk of disease deterioration.[80] For acute decompensated HF in the absence of ACS, cTnT is a prognostic marker for short-term and long-term outcomes.[81]

In addition, cTnI has been shown to reflect increased BNP levels, impaired hemodynamics, and worsening of left ventricular dysfunction.[82] For acute admissions, serial changes in cTnI levels over 90 days were functional in predicting increased likelihood of mortality and rehospitalization.[83] When used in combination with BNP measurements, cTnI measurements on admission were shown to predict in-hospital mortality, and increasing concentrations were associated with risk of death in a large-scale registry cohort (the Acute Decompensated Heart Failure National Registry [ADHERE]).[84,85]

Heart-Type Fatty Acid–Binding Protein

Heart-type fatty acid–binding protein (H-FABP) is a small cytosolic protein involved in transporting long-chain fatty acids in the myocardium and is released in response to myocardial damage,[86] indicating its potential as a sensitive biomarker for acute myocardial infarction (MI).[87] H-FABP concentrations are known to be increased in congestive and chronic HF,[88] and are reported to be more sensitive than troponin to detect myocardial damage and identify patients at high risk.[86] Initial investigations have been performed to understand the role and/or association of H-FABP in HF, but further studies are required to assess its utility in comparison with current clinical measurements.

C-Reactive Protein

C-reactive protein (CRP) is a traditional marker of inflammation and high concentrations are commonly associated with mortality in patients with acute MI. However, studies have also shown increased CRP levels in patients with HF, reflecting myocardial damage[89] and associations with HF severity, mortality and morbidity,[90] and rehospitalization.[91] Data indicate that CRP can be used as a predictor for deterioration of heart function;

however, it has also been reported to show no statistical association with left ventricular ejection fraction, providing complications for its suitability and specificity as a biomarker in HF.[92]

Tumor Necrosis Factor-α

Tumor necrosis factor-α (TNF-α) is a cytokine involved in inflammation and has been reported to be at increased levels in chronic HF.[93] TNF-α has also been implicated in patients with newly diagnosed HF, with increased levels associated with abnormal left atrial dysfunction, and advanced left ventricular diastolic and systolic dysfunction.[94] Further associations have been reported with NYHA class and disease severity,[95] along with the use of TNF-α as a predictor of mortality in advanced HF.[96]

Interleukin-6

IL-6 is also a cytokine involved in inflammation, but it has additional cardiovascular properties through regulation of cardiomyocyte hypertrophy and apoptosis.[97] Cardiac IL-6 expression is reported to increase in advanced HF, suggesting a potential role in prognosis.[98] In addition, increased IL-6 levels have been associated with left ventricular dysfunction before HF diagnosis, highlighting its potential utility as a risk marker for the onset and progression of HF.[99] This prognostic ability has been confirmed in acute HF for prediction of short-term and long-term mortality, both as a sole biomarker and in a multimarker approach when combined with NTproBNP.[100] Furthermore, IL-6, along with CRP and IL-4, concentrations have been shown to increase during a coronary event, returning to preevent levels as symptoms of HF subside over time. This observation indicates a potential role for IL-6 in differentiating between the decompensated and compensated states.[101]

MARKERS OF NEUROHORMONAL ACTIVATION
Copeptin

Preprovasopressin is proteolytically cleaved into copeptin, neurophysin II, and vasopressin, with the vasopressin also known as antidiuretic hormone, which has a prominent role in fluid homeostasis and has been shown to be related to the severity of HF.[102] However, vasopressin is known to show instability in circulation and therefore is troublesome for clinical measurements. In contrast, copeptin is considered to have high stability and is released in equimolar concentrations to vasopressin, allowing a more reliable and reproducible alternative for indirect measurement of vasopressin.[103] Initial research into the clinical role of copeptin as a prognostic biomarker has suggested it offers superiority over natriuretic peptides for prediction of 14-day and 90-day mortality in acute admissions[73,104] and longer-term prediction at 24 months for patients across various stages of disease,[105] as well as for those with advanced HF.[106] Although a contemporary biomarker for HF, data highlight copeptin measurements as a potential clinical tool for risk stratification, particularly in acute cases.

Matrix Metalloproteinases

Matrix metalloproteinases (MMPs) are a family of zinc-dependent protease enzymes required for normal tissue remodeling and mediating collagen metabolism and extracellular matrix (ECM) homeostasis.[107] Four common classes of MMPs have been identified: gelatinases (MMP-2 and MMP-9), collagenases (MMP-1 and MMP-8), stromelysin (MMP-3), and matrilysin (MMP-7), all of which are regulated by tissue inhibitors.[108]

Increased MMP-9 and MMP-2 concentrations have been reported in patients with HF,[105] with the latter associated with mortality.[109] In contrast, MMP-8 has been shown to have decreased concentrations in patients with chronic HF.[110] Although there are variable alterations of MMPs in patients and more extensive research is required to identify their individual suitability for prognostic investigation, data suggest that they offer additional information when included within a multibiomarker panel.[111] These panel risk scores can improve the information available to identify disease process and HF risk in line with changes to ECM collagen homeostasis and activity of enzymes of remodeling.

MARKERS OF REMODELING
Galectin-3

Galectin-3, a member of the lectin family, has been implicated in multiple aspects of HF physiology, including inflammation and ventricular remodeling. It is secreted by activated macrophages that proliferate and cause cardiac fibrosis,[112,113] and has been shown to provide a positive role as a prognostic marker of HF.[114,115] Increased gelactin-3 levels have been associated with an increased risk of HF and mortality,[116] with a 2-fold increase in levels associated with a 2-fold increase in risk of death or rehospitalization over an 18-month period.[114] Furthermore, increased concentrations have also been associated with adverse outcome in patients with HF with preserved ejection fraction (HFpEF).[117] As with many proteomic biomarkers of

HF, the role of gelactin-3 requires further research, but initial data suggest potential as a marker to stratify patients for HF with or without remodeling.

Growth Differentiation Factor-15

Growth differentiation factor-15 (GDF-15) is a stress-responsive, transforming growth factor beta-cytokine involved in inflammatory and apoptotic pathways of tissue injury. It is an emerging marker of cardiac dysfunction, and increased levels of GDF-15 have been shown to identify high-risk patients with cardiovascular disease.[118,119] Increased GDF-15 levels have shown mortality prediction in patients with chronic HF, with increased expression of GDF-15 linked to the promotion of protective mechanisms for inhibition of apoptosis, hypertrophy, and adverse remodeling.[120] Increased levels have also been reported to have prognostic utility in patients with both HF with reduced ejection fraction (HFrEF) and HFpEF, adding to current markers such as troponin and NTproBNP.[121,122] For acute decompensated HF, increased GDF-15 concentrations have shown prognostic value for predicting mortality and HF rehospitalization at 1 year, supported by 21 original studies.[123,124]

MARKERS OF ASSOCIATED COMORBIDITIES
Cystatin C

Cystatin C is a small protein molecule that is involved in the extracellular inhibition of cathepsins. It is removed from circulation through the kidneys, thus providing biomarker information for renal dysfunction and therefore an interest for cardiovascular disease.[125] Cystatin C has shown prognostic capabilities in patients with chronic HF as well as those with HFrEF.[126–128] These positive relationships with adverse outcome in HF, as well as providing information on dysfunction in the renal system, signify cystatin C as a useful biomarker for a combinatory view of cardiovascular disease and its comorbidities.

Neutrophil Gelatinase-Associated Lipocalin

Neutrophil gelatinase-associated lipocalin (NGAL) is an innate antibacterial factor protein of the lipocalin family, initially found to be expressed in neutrophils and later in kidney tubular cells. In kidney dysfunction, NGAL has been shown to be an early marker of injury in animal models and detectable in blood and urine following acute kidney injury.[129,130]

In patients with chronic HF, NGAL concentrations were found to be increased compared with healthy subjects.[131,132] However, their applicability as a prognostic marker was proved to be inferior to currently established protocols (eg, NTproBNP).[133] In acute cases, the GALLANT (NGAL Evaluation Along with B-type Natriuretic Peptide in acutely Decompensated Heart Failure) trial indicated that NGAL was a strong short-term (30 days) prognostic predictor of HF-related outcomes.[134]

Procalcitonin

Procalcitonin is a precursor peptide of calcitonin and a diagnostic marker of bacterial infections, such as in pneumonia,[135] with increased levels also measured in patients with HF.[136] Increased procalcitonin concentrations were able to predict the risk of long-term death and rehospitalization in acute admissions, irrespective of bacterial infections,[137] and were observed to be in line with disease severity for chronic patients.[138] In addition, serum procalcitonin concentrations provided diagnostic information for HF with high sensitivity and specificity.[139]

CONTEMPORARY PROTEOMIC BIOMARKERS

Recent research has led to an increased number of protein biomarkers that show promise in diagnosis and prognosis of HF conditions. For example, proenkephalin A (PENK) and chromogranin A (CgA) are proteins measured in the circulation that have shown utility as biomarkers in HF, and efforts to validate these for transition into a clinical setting are underway. PENK is a small endogenous opioid peptide that is cleaved to produce enkephalin. Studies have shown that enkephalins are released from nonneuronal tissues, including the kidneys and heart, in response to ischemia.[140] In chronic and acute HF, PENK is associated with glomerular function but does not offer significantly additive prognostic information in addition to current biomarkers of renal function.[141] However, it has provided useful prognostic information for hospitalization or mortality in patients with stable HF.[142] In addition, PENK concentrations have shown predictive capabilities for in-hospital mortality in patients with acute HF, as well as indicating patients at risk of worsening renal function.[143] CgA is a prohormone produced in various tissues, including the heart. Hyperglycosylations of CgA lead to its impaired conversion to catestatin, an action found to be associated with acute HF outcomes.[144] Mixed prognostic quality has been reported in the literature, with studies showing CgA to be associated with the severity of chronic HF and a prognostic marker for mortality,[145] but providing no additive information for

prognosis compared with established protocols and biomarkers.[146] In addition to CgA, chromogranin B, which is colocalized with CgA, has also shown an increase in concentrations to follow the severity and development of HF.[147]

Although PENK and CgA have been taken forward to extended validation studies, discovery-focused proteomics experiments have identified several circulating proteins as potential novel biomarkers for HF. The use of urine sampling as a less-invasive alternative to the traditional blood draw has led to an interest in highlighting urinary proteins for diagnostic testing in HF. Two proteins, insulinlike growth factor–binding protein 2 (IGFBP-2) and orosomucoid 1 (ORM1), have been reported to possess diagnostic potential, providing additive information to current biomarkers such as BNP for IGFBP-2,[148] as well as increasing concentrations in line with the severity of chronic HF and good diagnostic sensitivity (95%) and specificity (85%) for ORM1.[149] These proteins are examples of proteomic biomarkers that have provided initially positive associations, but further validation in extended experiments is required.

Other novel protein discoveries have been supported with initial mechanistic and/or clinical investigations and therefore are following the required pathway for translation into a clinical setting. Leucine-rich α2-glycoprotein (LRG) was reported to have an exaggerated expression in patients with a measured BNP of greater than or equal to 100 pg/mL and provided similar diagnostic statistics to BNP.[150] In addition to this, the investigators showed cardiac myocytes to be the origin of LRG release, and more recently it was observed that LRG was active in suppressing adverse remodeling post-MI,[151] and that LRG release in HF may be in response to pressure overload. Calcium-binding proteins A8/9 (S100A8/9) have also been reported to have an upregulated expression as a protective mechanism in HF development, with an observed contribution to the anti-HF effect of hypertrophic preconditioning.[152] In addition to their mechanistic interactions, S100A8/9 have also been shown to provide predictive qualities for mortality in elder patients with severe HF.[153] Similarly, levels of circulating heat shock protein 70 (HSP70) have been shown to increase concurrently with cardiac expression[154] and HF severity,[155] and HSP70 has been implicated as a potential biomarker for early diagnosis of HF.[155]

Although the prior examples of novel biomarkers have undergone initial stages of mechanistic and clinical validation, more recent experiments have indicated further potential biomarkers that remain at the discovery phase. For example, quiescin

Q6 (QSOX1) has shown promise as a biomarker that is specific to acute decompensated HF with dyspnea, with reduced and comparable levels measured in patients with chronic HF and healthy volunteers.[156] QSOX1 has been shown to increase in the left ventricle in an animal HF model[157] and provides diagnostic qualities that are equal to those of BNP and NTproBNP,[156] with increased specificity compared with natriuretic peptides for diagnosis of acute decompensated HF, irrespective of the presence of previous stable HF.

Many candidate proteomic biomarkers for HF have been discovered and are still in the research phase to determine their roles in HF. Limited information regarding their additive role as biomarkers in HF is available and further research for their capacity is required. Extending from single biomarker analyses, proteome-wide investigations have provided insight into multibiomarker models to predict future disease developments. A notable example was presented by Hollander and colleagues,[158] who identified a list of 17 candidate protein biomarkers that, when combined with BNP measurements, were able to provide 97% sensitivity and 100% specificity for classifying patients on recovery from cardiac transplants. This finding provides an opportunity to provide outpatient screening to monitor response to HF treatments but requires extensive additional testing to validate its applicability for everyday clinical use.

SUMMARY

A wide range of protein-based cardiac biomarkers have shown success in diagnostic and prognostic applications, with several already established as routine measurements in clinical laboratories. Extensive research efforts are currently underway to enhance the current knowledge of protein–cardiovascular disease interactions, led by proteomic-based organizations such as Human Proteome Organization (HUPO). The flagship venture has been The Human Proteome Project (HPP), which is working to map the entire human proteome to further understanding of the localized and systems biology of proteins and protein-protein interactions for diagnostic, prognostic, and therapeutic roles in disease.[2] In particular, HUPO has emphasized the need to develop open-access databases that allow the sharing of proteomics research data across equipment and institutions to detail the human proteome library.[159]

The advancement of technologies, such as MS, that complement traditional enzyme-based assays has allowed the development of highly sensitive and selective methods with the ability to measure multiple relevant biomarkers in a high-throughput manner. Although at a stage of infancy for translation to functional clinical laboratories, these methods offer the potential for future advancements in the breadth and depth of clinically relevant biomarkers. In addition, the use of multiple omics-based investigatory pathways, including proteomics, metabolomics, lipidomics, and genomics, may lead to the discovery and validation of novel biomarkers that provide improved clinical information to patients in cardiovascular disease and beyond. An example of this approach includes the focus of implementing the combination of protein and metabolite biomarkers to improve risk stratification, with recent demonstration of enhanced prognostic capabilities in chronic and acute HF when combining BNP/NTproBNP with trimethylamine N-oxide, a metabolite biomarker linked to gut microbial breakdown of dietary molecules.[160,161] Continued efforts for biomarker discovery and validation promise to unearth novel and contemporary molecules for application in personalized and precision medicine, with the potential to lead to improved prognosis, treatment, and early diagnosis of conditions at the center of public health concerns.

REFERENCES

1. Jensen ON. Modification-specific proteomics: characterization of post-translational modifications by mass spectrometry. Curr Opin Chem Biol 2004;8:33–41.
2. Legrain P, Aebersold R, Archakov A, et al. The human proteome project: current state and future direction. Mol Cell Proteomics 2011;10. M111. 009993.
3. Chan D, Ng LL. Biomarkers in acute myocardial infarction. BMC Med 2010;8:34.
4. Maisel AS, Krishnaswamy P, Nowak RM, et al. Rapid measurement of B-type natriuretic peptide in the emergency diagnosis of heart failure. N Engl J Med 2002;347:161–7.
5. Newby LK, Christenson RH, Ohman EM, et al. Value of serial troponin T measures for early and late risk stratification in patients with acute coronary syndromes. Circulation 1998;98:1853–9.
6. Strimbu K, Tavel JA. What are biomarkers? Curr Opin HIV AIDS 2010;5:463.
7. Mayeux R. Biomarkers: potential uses and limitations. NeuroRx 2004;1:182–8.
8. Cowie MR, Jourdain P, Maisel A, et al. Clinical applications of B-type natriuretic peptide (BNP) testing. Eur Heart J 2003;24:1710–8.
9. Roger VL. Epidemiology of heart failure. Circ Res 2013;113:646–59.

10. Mentz RJ, O'Connor CM. Pathophysiology and clinical evaluation of acute heart failure. Nat Rev Cardiol 2016;13:28–35.

11. Bui AL, Horwich TB, Fonarow GC. Epidemiology and risk profile of heart failure. Nat Rev Cardiol 2011;8:30–41.

12. Yancy CW, Jessup M, Bozkurt B, et al. 2013 ACCF/AHA guideline for the management of heart failure. Circulation 2013;128:e240–327.

13. Li W, Rong R, Zhao S, et al. Proteomic analysis of metabolic, cytoskeletal and stress response proteins in human heart failure. J Cell Mol Med 2012; 16:59–71.

14. James P. Protein identification in the post-genome era: the rapid rise of proteomics. Q Rev Biophys 1997;30:279–331.

15. Graves PR, Haystead TA. Molecular biologist's guide to proteomics. Microbiol Mol Biol Rev 2002; 66:39–63.

16. Schiess R, Wollscheid B, Aebersold R. Targeted proteomic strategy for clinical biomarker discovery. Mol Oncol 2009;3:33–44.

17. Zhou W, Petricoin EF, Longo C. Mass spectrometry-based biomarker discovery. Methods Mol Biol 2012;823:251–64.

18. Hathout Y. Proteomic methods for biomarker discovery and validation. Are we there yet? Expert Rev Proteomics 2015;12:329–31.

19. Schoenhoff FS, Fu Q, Van Eyk JE. Cardiovascular proteomics: implications for clinical applications. Clin Lab Med 2009;29:87–99.

20. Melanson JE, Chisholm KA, Pinto DM. Targeted comparative proteomics by liquid chromatography/matrix-assisted laser desorption/ionization triple-quadrupole mass spectrometry. Rapid Commun Mass Spectrom 2006;20:904–10.

21. Carr SA, Abbatiello SE, Ackermann BL, et al. Targeted peptide measurements in biology and medicine: best practices for mass spectrometry-based assay development using a fit-for-purpose approach. Mol Cell Proteomics 2014;13:907–17.

22. Pan S, Aebersold R, Chen R, et al. Mass spectrometry based targeted protein quantification: methods and applications. J Proteome Res 2008; 8:787–97.

23. Mbasu RJ, Heaney LM, Molloy BJ, et al. Advances in quadrupole and time-of-flight mass spectrometry for peptide MRM based translational research analysis. Proteomics 2016;16:2206–20.

24. Pan S, Zhang H, Rush J, et al. High throughput proteome screening for biomarker detection. Mol Cell Proteomics 2005;4:182–90.

25. Pan S, Rush J, Peskind ER, et al. Application of targeted quantitative proteomics analysis in human cerebrospinal fluid using a liquid chromatography matrix-assisted laser desorption/ionization time-of-flight tandem mass spectrometer (LC MALDI TOF/TOF) platform. J Proteome Res 2008;7:720–30.

26. Reyzer ML, Caprioli RM. MALDI mass spectrometry for direct tissue analysis: a new tool for biomarker discovery. J Proteome Res 2005;4: 1138–42.

27. Suzuki T, Israr MZ, Heaney LM, et al. Prognostic role of molecular forms of B-type natriuretic peptide in acute heart failure. Clin Chem 2017;63: 880–6.

28. Rifai N, Gillette MA, Carr SA. Protein biomarker discovery and validation: the long and uncertain path to clinical utility. Nat Biotechnol 2006;24:971–83.

29. Heaney LM, Jones DJL, Suzuki T. Mass spectrometry in medicine: a technology for the future? Future Sci OA 2017;3:FSO213. http://dx.doi.org/10.4155/fsoa-2017-0053.

30. Vasan RS. Biomarkers of cardiovascular disease. Circulation 2006;113:2335–62.

31. Levin ER, Gardner DG, Samson WK. Natriuretic peptides. N Engl J Med 1998;339:321–8.

32. Correa de Sa DD, Chen HH. The role of natriuretic peptides in heart failure. Curr Heart Fail Rep 2008; 5:177–84.

33. Dao Q, Krishnaswamy P, Kazanegra R, et al. Utility of B-type natriuretic peptide in the diagnosis of congestive heart failure in an urgent-care setting. J Am Coll Cardiol 2001;37:379–85.

34. Cowie MR, Struthers AD, Wood DA, et al. Value of natriuretic peptides in assessment of patients with possible new heart failure in primary care. Lancet 1997;350:1349–53.

35. McCullough PA, Nowak RM, McCord J, et al. B-type natriuretic peptide and clinical judgment in emergency diagnosis of heart failure. Circulation 2002;106:416–22.

36. Jourdain P, Jondeau G, Funck F, et al. Plasma brain natriuretic peptide-guided therapy to improve outcome in heart failure: the STARS-BNP Multicenter Study. J Am Coll Cardiol 2007; 49:1733–9.

37. Doust JA, Pietrzak E, Dobson A, et al. How well does B-type natriuretic peptide predict death and cardiac events in patients with heart failure: systematic review. BMJ 2005;330:625.

38. Cheng V, Kazanegra R, Garcia A, et al. A rapid bedside test for B-type peptide predicts treatment outcomes in patients admitted for decompensated heart failure: a pilot study. J Am Coll Cardiol 2001; 37:386–91.

39. Luchner A, Burnett JC Jr, Jougasaki M, et al. Evaluation of brain natriuretic peptide as marker of left ventricular dysfunction and hypertrophy in the population. J Hypertens 2000;18:1121–8.

40. Maisel A, Mueller C, Adams K, et al. State of the art: using natriuretic peptide levels in clinical practice. Eur J Heart Fail 2008;10:824–39.

41. Felker GM, Hasselblad V, Hernandez AF, et al. Biomarker-guided therapy in chronic heart failure: a meta analysis of randomized controlled trials. Am Heart J 2009;158:422–30.

42. Ewald B, Ewald D, Thakkinstian A, et al. Meta-analysis of B type natriuretic peptide and N-terminal pro B natriuretic peptide in the diagnosis of clinical heart failure and population screening for left ventricular systolic dysfunction. Intern Med J 2008; 38:101–13.

43. Januzzi JL, van Kimmenade R, Lainchbury J, et al. NT-proBNP testing for diagnosis and short-term prognosis in acute destabilized heart failure: an international pooled analysis of 1256 patients. Eur Heart J 2006;27:330–7.

44. Potter LR. Natriuretic peptide metabolism, clearance and degradation. FEBS J 2011;278:1808–17.

45. Mueller T, Gegenhuber A, Dieplinger B, et al. Long-term stability of endogenous B-type natriuretic peptide (BNP) and amino terminal proBNP (NT-proBNP) in frozen plasma samples. Clin Chem Lab Med 2004;42:942–4.

46. Gustafsson F, Steensgaard-Hansen F, Badskjær J, et al. Diagnostic and prognostic performance of N-terminal ProBNP in primary care patients with suspected heart failure. J Card Fail 2005;11:S15–20.

47. McDonagh TA, Holmer S, Raymond I, et al. NT-proBNP and the diagnosis of heart failure: a pooled analysis of three European epidemiological studies. Eur J Heart Fail 2004;6:269–73.

48. Ozturk TC, Unluer E, Denizbasi A, et al. Can NT-proBNP be used as a criterion for heart failure hospitalization in emergency room? J Res Med Sci 2011;16:1564.

49. Taylor CJ, Roalfe AK, Iles R, et al. The potential role of NT-proBNP in screening for and predicting prognosis in heart failure: a survival analysis. BMJ 2014; 4:e004675.

50. Lainchbury JG, Troughton RW, Strangman KM, et al. N-terminal pro–B-type natriuretic peptide-guided treatment for chronic heart failure: results from the BATTLESCARRED (NT-proBNP–Assisted Treatment To Lessen Serial Cardiac Readmissions and Death) trial. J Am Coll Cardiol 2009;55:53–60.

51. Bettencourt P. NT-proBNP and BNP: biomarkers for heart failure management. Eur J Heart Fail 2004;6: 359–63.

52. Seino Y, Ogawa A, Yamashita T, et al. Application of NT-proBNP and BNP measurements in cardiac care: a more discerning marker for the detection and evaluation of heart failure. Eur J Heart Fail 2004;6:295–300.

53. Roberts E, Ludman AJ, Dworzynski K, et al. The diagnostic accuracy of the natriuretic peptides in heart failure: systematic review and diagnostic meta-analysis in the acute care setting. BMJ 2015;350:h910.

54. Kim HN, Januzzi JL. Natriuretic peptide testing in heart failure. Circulation 2011;123:2015–9.

55. Masson S, Latini R, Anand IS, et al. Direct comparison of B-type natriuretic peptide (BNP) and amino-terminal proBNP in a large population of patients with chronic and symptomatic heart failure: the Valsartan Heart Failure (Val-HeFT) data. Clin Chem 2006;52:1528–38.

56. Niederkofler EE, Kiernan UA, O'Rear J, et al. Detection of endogenous B-type natriuretic peptide at very low concentrations in patients with heart failure. Circ Heart Fail 2008;1:258–64.

57. Fujimoto H, Suzuki T, Aizawa K, et al. Processed B-type natriuretic peptide is a biomarker of postinterventional restenosis in ischemic heart disease. Clin Chem 2013;59:1330–7.

58. Miller WL, Phelps MA, Wood CM, et al. Comparison of mass spectrometry and clinical assay measurements of circulating fragments of B-type natriuretic peptide in patients with chronic heart failure. Circ Heart Fail 2011;4:355–60.

59. Tsutamoto T, Wada A, Maeda K, et al. Attenuation of compensation of endogenous cardiac natriuretic peptide system in chronic heart failure. Circulation 1997;96:509–16.

60. Clerico A, Iervasi G, Del Chicca MG, et al. Circulating levels of cardiac natriuretic peptides (ANP and BNP) measured by highly sensitive and specific immunoradiometric assays in normal subjects and in patients with different degrees of heart failure. J Endocrinol Invest 1998;21:170–9.

61. Luers C, Sutcliffe A, Binder L, et al. NT-proANP and NT-proBNP as prognostic markers in patients with acute decompensated heart failure of different etiologies. Clin Biochem 2013;46:1013–9.

62. Lerman A, Gibbons RJ, Rodeheffer RJ, et al. Circulating N-terminal atrial natriuretic peptide as a marker for symptomless left-ventricular dysfunction. Lancet 1993;341:1105–9.

63. Maisel A, Mueller C, Nowak R, et al. Mid-region pro-hormone markers for diagnosis and prognosis in acute dyspnea: results from the BACH (Biomarkers in Acute Heart Failure) trial. J Am Coll Cardiol 2010;55:2062–76.

64. von Haehling S, Jankowska EA, Morgenthaler NG, et al. Comparison of midregional pro-atrial natriuretic peptide with N-terminal pro-B-type natriuretic peptide in predicting survival in patients with chronic heart failure. J Am Coll Cardiol 2007; 50:1973–80.

65. Gegenhuber A, Struck J, Poelz W, et al. Midregional pro-A-type natriuretic peptide measurements for diagnosis of acute destabilized heart failure in short-of-breath patients: comparison with B-type natriuretic peptide (BNP) and amino-terminal proBNP. Clin Chem 2006;52:827–31.

66. Sanada S, Hakuno D, Higgins LJ, et al. IL-33 and ST2 comprise a critical biomechanically induced and cardioprotective signaling system. J Clin Invest 2007;117:1538–49.

67. Weinberg EO, Shimpo M, Hurwitz S, et al. Identification of serum soluble ST2 receptor as a novel heart failure biomarker. Circulation 2003;107:721–6.

68. Rehman SU, Mueller T, Januzzi JL. Characteristics of the novel interleukin family biomarker ST2 in patients with acute heart failure. J Am Coll Cardiol 2008;52:1458–65.

69. Januzzi JL, Peacock WF, Maisel AS, et al. Measurement of the interleukin family member ST2 in patients with acute dyspnea. J Am Coll Cardiol 2007;50:607–13.

70. Jougasaki M, Rodeheffer RJ, Redfield MM, et al. Cardiac secretion of adrenomedullin in human heart failure. J Clin Invest 1996;97:2370.

71. Peacock WF. Novel biomarkers in acute heart failure: MR-pro-adrenomedullin. Clin Chem Lab Med 2014;52:1433–5.

72. Lassus J, Gayat E, Mueller C, et al. Incremental value of biomarkers to clinical variables for mortality prediction in acutely decompensated heart failure: the Multinational Observational Cohort on Acute Heart Failure (MOCA) study. Int J Cardiol 2013;168:2186–94.

73. Frank Peacock W, Nowak R, Christenson R, et al. Short-term mortality risk in emergency department acute heart failure. Acad Emerg Med 2011;18:947–58.

74. Wang TJ. Significance of circulating troponins in heart failure. Circulation 2007;116:1217–20.

75. Missov E, Calzolari C, Pau B. Circulating cardiac troponin I in severe congestive heart failure. Circulation 1997;96:2953–8.

76. Missov E, Mair J. A novel biochemical approach to congestive heart failure: cardiac troponin T. Am Heart J 1999;138:95–9.

77. Latini R, Masson S, Anand IS, et al. Prognostic value of very low plasma concentrations of troponin T in patients with stable chronic heart failure. Circulation 2007;116:1242–9.

78. Setsuta K, Seino Y, Takahashi N, et al. Clinical significance of elevated levels of cardiac troponin T in patients with chronic heart failure. Am J Cardiol 1999;84:608–11.

79. Ishii J, Cui W, Kitagawa F, et al. Prognostic value of combination of cardiac troponin T and B-type natriuretic peptide after initiation of treatment in patients with chronic heart failure. Clin Chem 2003;49:2020–6.

80. Perna ER, Macin SM, Canella JP, et al. Ongoing myocardial injury in stable severe heart failure. Circulation 2004;110:2376–82.

81. Sakhuja R, Green S, Oestreicher EM, et al. Amino-terminal pro–brain natriuretic peptide, brain natriuretic peptide, and troponin t for prediction of mortality in acute heart failure. Clin Chem 2007;53:412–20.

82. Horwich TB, Patel J, MacLellan WR, et al. Cardiac troponin I is associated with impaired hemodynamics, progressive left ventricular dysfunction, and increased mortality rates in advanced heart failure. Circulation 2003;108:833–8.

83. Xue Y, Clopton P, Peacock WF, et al. Serial changes in high-sensitive troponin I predict outcome in patients with decompensated heart failure. Eur J Heart Fail 2011;13:37–42.

84. Fonarow GC, Peacock WF, Horwich TB, et al. Usefulness of B-type natriuretic peptide and cardiac troponin levels to predict in-hospital mortality from ADHERE. Am J Cardiol 2008;101:231–7.

85. Peacock WF IV, De Marco T, Fonarow GC, et al. Cardiac troponin and outcome in acute heart failure. N Engl J Med 2008;358:2117–26.

86. Niizeki T, Takeishi Y, Arimoto T, et al. Heart-type fatty acid-binding protein is more sensitive than troponin T to detect the ongoing myocardial damage in chronic heart failure patients. J Card Fail 2007;13:120–7.

87. Lili C, Xiaomei G, Fei Y. Role of heart-type fatty acid binding protein in early detection of acute myocardial infarction in comparison with cTnI, CK-MB and myoglobin. J Huazhong Univ Sci Technolog Med Sci 2004;24:449–51.

88. Arimoto T, Takeishi Y, Shiga R, et al. Prognostic value of elevated circulating heart-type fatty acid binding protein in patients with congestive heart failure. J Card Fail 2005;11:56–60.

89. Berton G, Cordiano R, Palmieri R, et al. C-reactive protein in acute myocardial infarction: association with heart failure. Am Heart J 2003;145:1094–101.

90. Anand IS, Latini R, Florea VG, et al. C-reactive protein in heart failure. Circulation 2005;112:1428–34.

91. Alonso-Martinez JL, Llorente-Diez B, Echegaray-Agara M, et al. C-reactive protein as a predictor of improvement and readmission in heart failure. Eur J Heart Fail 2002;4:331–6.

92. Oikonomou E, Tousoulis DI, Siasos GE, et al. The role of inflammation in heart failure: new therapeutic approaches. Hellenic J Cardiol 2011;52:30–40.

93. Levine B, Kalman J, Mayer L, et al. Elevated circulating levels of tumor necrosis factor in severe chronic heart failure. N Engl J Med 1990;323:236–41.

94. Chrysohoou C, Pitsavos C, Barbetseas J, et al. Chronic systemic inflammation accompanies impaired ventricular diastolic function, detected by Doppler imaging, in patients with newly diagnosed systolic heart failure (Hellenic Heart Failure Study). Heart Vessels 2009;24:22–6.

95. Rivera M, Taléns-Visconti R, Sirera R, et al. Soluble TNF-α and interleukin-6 receptors in the urine of heart failure patients. Their clinical value and

relationship with plasma levels. Eur J Heart Fail 2004;6:877–82.

96. Deswal A, Petersen NJ, Feldman AM, et al. Cytokines and cytokine receptors in advanced heart failure. Circulation 2001;103:2055–9.

97. Wollert KC, Drexler H. The role of interleukin-6 in the failing heart. Heart Fail Rev 2001;6:95–103.

98. Gabriele P, Zhi Fang S, Tonny DT, et al. Activation of the cardiac interleukin-6 system in advanced heart failure. Eur J Heart Fail 2001;3:415–21.

99. Raymond RJ, Dehmer GJ, Theoharides TC, et al. Elevated interleukin-6 levels in patients with asymptomatic left ventricular systolic dysfunction. Am Heart J 2001;141:435–8.

100. Pudil R, Tichý M, Andrýs C, et al. Plasma interleukin-6 level is associated with NT-proBNP level and predicts short-and long-term mortality in patients with acute heart failure. Acta Medica (Hradec Kralove) 2010;53:225–8.

101. Sato Y, Takatsu Y, Kataoka K, et al. Serial circulating concentrations of C-reactive protein, interleukin (IL)-4, and IL-6 in patients with acute left heart decompensation. Clin Cardiol 1999;22:811–3.

102. Nakamura T, Funayama H, Yoshimura A, et al. Possible vascular role of increased plasma arginine vasopressin in congestive heart failure. Int J Cardiol 2006;106:191–5.

103. Morgenthaler NG, Struck J, Alonso C, et al. Assay for the measurement of copeptin, a stable peptide derived from the precursor of vasopressin. Clin Chem 2006;52:112–9.

104. Maisel A, Xue Y, Shah K, et al. Increased 90-day mortality in patients with acute heart failure with elevated copeptin: secondary results from the Biomarkers in Acute Heart Failure (BACH) study. Circ Heart Fail 2011;4:613–20.

105. Neuhold S, Huelsmann M, Strunk G, et al. Comparison of copeptin, B-type natriuretic peptide, and amino-terminal pro-B-type natriuretic peptide in patients with chronic heart failure: prediction of death at different stages of the disease. J Am Coll Cardiol 2008;52:266–72.

106. Stoiser B, Mörtl D, Hülsmann M, et al. Copeptin, a fragment of the vasopressin precursor, as a novel predictor of outcome in heart failure. Eur J Clin Invest 2006;36:771–8.

107. Spinale FG. Myocardial matrix remodeling and the matrix metalloproteinases: influence on cardiac form and function. Physiol Rev 2007;87:1285–342.

108. Yamazaki T, Lee JD, Shimizu H, et al. Circulating matrix metalloproteinase-2 is elevated in patients with congestive heart failure. Eur J Heart Fail 2004;6:41–5.

109. George J, Patal S, Wexler D, et al. Circulating matrix metalloproteinase-2 but not matrix metalloproteinase-3, matrix metalloproteinase-9, or tissue inhibitor of metalloproteinase-1 predicts outcome in patients with congestive heart failure. Am Heart J 2005;150:484–7.

110. Wilson EM, Gunasinghe HR, Coker ML, et al. Plasma matrix metalloproteinase and inhibitor profiles in patients with heart failure. J Card Fail 2002;8:390–8.

111. Zile MR, DeSantis SM, Baicu CF, et al. Plasma biomarkers that reflect determinants of matrix composition identify the presence of left ventricular hypertrophy and diastolic heart failure. Circ Heart Fail 2011;4:246–56.

112. McCullough PA, Olobatoke A, Vanhecke TE. Galectin-3: a novel blood test for the evaluation and management of patients with heart failure. Rev Cardiovasc Med 2010;12:200–10.

113. Lin YH, Lin LY, Wu YW, et al. The relationship between serum galectin-3 and serum markers of cardiac extracellular matrix turnover in heart failure patients. Clin Chim Acta 2009;409:96–9.

114. Lok DJ, Van Der Meer P, Lipsic E, et al. Prognostic value of galectin-3, a novel marker of fibrosis, in patients with chronic heart failure: data from the DEAL-HF study. Clin Res Cardiol 2010;99:323–8.

115. Grandin EW, Jarolim P, Murphy SA, et al. Galectin-3 and the development of heart failure after acute coronary syndrome: pilot experience from PROVE IT-TIMI 22. Clin Chem 2012;58:267–73.

116. Ho JE, Liu C, Lyass A, et al. Galectin-3, a marker of cardiac fibrosis, predicts incident heart failure in the community. J Am Coll Cardiol 2012;60:1249–56.

117. Edelmann F, Holzendorf V, Wachter R, et al. Galectin-3 in patients with heart failure with preserved ejection fraction: results from the Aldo-DHF trial. Eur J Heart Fail 2015;17:214–23.

118. Kempf T, Wollert KC. Growth differentiation factor-15: a new biomarker in cardiovascular disease. Herz 2009;34:594–9.

119. Wollert KC, Kempf T. Growth differentiation factor 15 in heart failure: an update. Curr Heart Fail Rep 2012;9:337–45.

120. Kempf T, von Haehling S, Peter T, et al. Prognostic utility of growth differentiation factor-15 in patients with chronic heart failure. J Am Coll Cardiol 2007;50:1054–60.

121. de Boer RA, Lok DJ, Jaarsma T, et al. Predictive value of plasma galectin-3 levels in heart failure with reduced and preserved ejection fraction. Ann Med 2011;43:60–8.

122. Chan MM, Santhanakrishnan R, Chong JP, et al. Growth differentiation factor 15 in heart failure with preserved vs. reduced ejection fraction. Eur J Heart Fail 2016;18:81–8.

123. Jankovic-Tomasevic R, Pavlovic SU, Jevtovic-Stoimenov T, et al. Prognostic utility of biomarker growth differentiation factor-15 in patients with

acute decompensated heart failure. Acta Cardiol 2016;71:587–95.

124. George M, Jena A, Srivatsan V, et al. GDF 15-A novel biomarker in the offing for heart failure. Curr Cardiol Rev 2016;12:37–46.

125. Angelidis C, Deftereos S, Giannopoulos G, et al. Cystatin C: an emerging biomarker in cardiovascular disease. Curr Top Med Chem 2013;13:164–79.

126. Huerta A, López B, Ravassa S, et al. Association of cystatin C with heart failure with preserved ejection fraction in elderly hypertensive patients: potential role of altered collagen metabolism. J Hypertens 2016;34:130–8.

127. Carrasco-Sánchez FJ, Galisteo-Almeda L, Páez-Rubio I, et al. Prognostic value of cystatin C on admission in heart failure with preserved ejection fraction. J Card Fail 2011;17:31–8.

128. Nosaka K, Nakamura K, Kusano K, et al. Serum cystatin C as a biomarker of cardiac diastolic dysfunction in patients with cardiac disease and preserved ejection fraction. Congest Heart Fail 2013;19:E35–9.

129. Devarajan P. Neutrophil gelatinase-associated lipocalin (NGAL): a new marker of kidney disease. Scand J Clin Lab Invest Suppl 2008;68:89–94.

130. Mishra J, Ma Q, Prada A, et al. Identification of neutrophil gelatinase-associated lipocalin as a novel early urinary biomarker for ischemic renal injury. J Am Soc Nephrol 2003;14:2534–43.

131. Yndestad A, Landrø L, Ueland T, et al. Increased systemic and myocardial expression of neutrophil gelatinase-associated lipocalin in clinical and experimental heart failure. Eur Heart J 2009;30: 1229–36.

132. Aghel A, Shrestha K, Mullens W, et al. Serum neutrophil gelatinase-associated lipocalin (NGAL) in predicting worsening renal function in acute decompensated heart failure. J Card Fail 2010;16:49–54.

133. Nymo SH, Ueland T, Askevold ET, et al. The association between neutrophil gelatinase-associated lipocalin and clinical outcome in chronic heart failure: results from CORONA. J Intern Med 2012;271: 436–43.

134. Maisel AS, Mueller C, Fitzgerald R, et al. Prognostic utility of plasma neutrophil gelatinase-associated lipocalin in patients with acute heart failure: the NGAL EvaLuation Along with B-type NaTriuretic Peptide in acutely decompensated heart failure (GALLANT) trial. Eur J Heart Fail 2011;13:846–51.

135. Christ-Crain M, Jaccard-Stolz D, Bingisser R, et al. Effect of procalcitonin-guided treatment on antibiotic use and outcome in lower respiratory tract infections: cluster-randomised, single-blinded intervention trial. Lancet 2004;363:600–7.

136. Maisel A, Neath SX, Landsberg J, et al. Use of procalcitonin for the diagnosis of pneumonia in

patients presenting with a chief complaint of dyspnoea: results from the BACH (Biomarkers in Acute Heart Failure) trial. Eur J Heart Fail 2012;14:278–86.

137. Villanueva MP, Mollar A, Palau P, et al. Procalcitonin and long-term prognosis after an admission for acute heart failure. Eur J Intern Med 2015;26:42–8.

138. Wang W, Zhang X, Ge N, et al. Procalcitonin testing for diagnosis and short-term prognosis in bacterial infection complicated by congestive heart failure: a multicenter analysis of 4,698 cases. Crit Care 2014; 18:R4.

139. Canbay A, Celebi OO, Celebi S, et al. Procalcitonin: a marker of heart failure. Acta Cardiol 2015; 70:473–8.

140. Denning GM, Ackermann LW, Barna TJ, et al. Proenkephalin expression and enkephalin release are widely observed in non-neuronal tissues. Peptides 2008;29:83–92.

141. Matsue Y, ter Maaten JM, Struck J, et al. Clinical correlates and prognostic value of proenkephalin in acute and chronic heart failure. J Card Fail 2017;23:231–9.

142. Arbit B, Marston N, Shah K, et al. Prognostic usefulness of proenkephalin in stable ambulatory patients with heart failure. Am J Cardiol 2016;117: 1310–4.

143. Ng LL, Squire IB, Jones DJ, et al. Proenkephalin, renal dysfunction, and prognosis in patients with acute heart failure: a GREAT network study. J Am Coll Cardiol 2017;69:56–69.

144. Ottesen AH, Carlson CR, Louch WE, et al. Glycosylated chromogranin A in heart failure: implications for processing and cardiomyocyte calcium homeostasis. Circ Heart Fail 2017;10:e003675.

145. Ceconi C, Ferrari R, Bachetti T, et al. Chromogranin A in heart failure; a novel neurohumoral factor and a predictor for mortality. Eur Heart J 2002;23: 967–74.

146. Røsjø H, Masson S, Latini R, et al. Prognostic value of chromogranin A in chronic heart failure: data from the GISSI-Heart Failure trial. Eur J Heart Fail 2010;12:549–56.

147. Røsjø H, Husberg C, Dahl MB, et al. Chromogranin B in heart failure: a putative cardiac biomarker expressed in the failing myocardium. Circ Heart Fail 2010;3:503–11.

148. Berry M, Galinier M, Delmas C, et al. Proteomics analysis reveals IGFBP2 as a candidate diagnostic biomarker for heart failure. IJC Metab Endocr 2015; 6:5–12.

149. Hou LN, Li F, Zeng QC, et al. Excretion of urinary orosomucoid 1 protein is elevated in patients with chronic heart failure. PLoS One 2014;9:e107550.

150. Watson CJ, Ledwidge MT, Phelan D, et al. Proteomic analysis of coronary sinus serum reveals leucine-rich α2-glycoprotein as a novel biomarker

of ventricular dysfunction and heart failure. Circ Heart Fail 2011;4:188–97.

151. Kumagai S, Nakayama H, Fujimoto M, et al. Myeloid cell-derived LRG attenuates adverse cardiac remodelling after myocardial infarction. Cardiovasc Res 2016;109:272–82.

152. Wei X, Wu B, Zhao J, et al. Myocardial hypertrophic preconditioning attenuates cardiomyocyte hypertrophy and slows progression to heart failure through upregulation of S100A8/A9. Circulation 2015;131:1506–17.

153. Ma LP, Haugen E, Ikemoto M, et al. S100A8/A9 complex as a new biomarker in prediction of mortality in elderly patients with severe heart failure. Int J Cardiol 2012;155:26–32.

154. Wei YJ, Huang YX, Shen Y, et al. Proteomic analysis reveals significant elevation of heat shock protein 70 in patients with chronic heart failure due to arrhythmogenic right ventricular cardiomyopathy. Mol Cell Biochem 2009;332:103–11.

155. Li Z, Song Y, Xing R, et al. Heat shock protein 70 acts as a potential biomarker for early diagnosis of heart failure. PLoS One 2013;8:e67964.

156. Mebazaa A, Vanpoucke G, Thomas G, et al. Unbiased plasma proteomics for novel diagnostic biomarkers in cardiovascular disease: identification of quiescin Q6 as a candidate biomarker of acutely decompensated heart failure. Eur Heart J 2012;33: 2317–24.

157. Toischer K, Rokita AG, Unsöld B, et al. Differential cardiac remodeling in preload versus afterload. Circulation 2010;122:993–1003.

158. Hollander Z, Lazárová M, Lam KK, et al. Proteomic biomarkers of recovered heart function. Eur J Heart Fail 2014;16:551–9.

159. Orchard S, Hermjakob H, Apweiler R. The proteomics standards initiative. Proteomics 2003;3: 1374–6.

160. Tang WW, Wang Z, Fan Y, et al. Prognostic value of elevated levels of intestinal microbe-generated metabolite trimethylamine-N-oxide in patients with heart failure. J Am Coll Cardiol 2014;64:1908–14.

161. Suzuki T, Heaney LM, Bhandari SS, et al. Trimethylamine N-oxide and prognosis in acute heart failure. Heart 2016;102:841–8.

Metabolic Biomarkers in Heart Failure

Chonyang L. Albert, MD[a], W.H. Wilson Tang, MD[a,b],*

KEYWORDS

- Heart failure metabolomics • Arginine • Nitric oxide • Myocardial energy utilization • Acylcarnitine
- TMAO

KEY POINTS

- Metabolomics is the study of small, organic, molecules of biochemical pathways, some of which are strongly implicated in heart failure pathogenesis and progression.
- Modern developments in mass spectrometry and nuclear magnetic resonance (NMR) have enabled identification of approximately 40,000 human metabolites.
- The failing heart exhibits metabolic derangements, particularly in energy utilization and oxidation.
- Creation of metabolomic profiles may aid in the diagnosis, management, and prognosis of heart failure.
- Metabolomics extends to human and microbial products, further adding to the complex gene, protein, and environmental interactions in heart failure.

INTRODUCTION

Heart failure is a complex disease process that affects an increasing number of patients due to advancements in cardiac care and increased longevity of the aging population. From an epidemiologic and macroscopic perspective, timely diagnosis and early interventions in heart failure are likely to have far-reaching impact on health care economics and public health. Many discoveries in pathophysiology and pharmacotherapy have already improved mortality and morbidity in this population of patients in the past few decades. However, for all the progress in the diagnosis and management of this complex disease, there remain many unresolved mysteries, the unlocking of which could lead to profound understanding of heart failure pathogenesis, treatment, and prognosis. From a microscopic perspective, heart failure is a manifestation of metabolic derangements on the cellular, genetic, proteomic, and metabolic levels.[1]

Traditionally, genetic information is translated from DNA into RNA and transcribed into protein. The proteome is made of a variety of proteins that can then undergo posttranscription modification, and through interactions with environmental factors, produce metabolites used for energy production. A metabolite is thus defined as any small organic molecule detectable in the human body with a molecular weight of 50 to 1500 Da. The source of metabolite generation can include any biofluid, such as blood, urine, saliva, and respiratory gases. Thus, a rich collection of metabolites, including peptides, oligonucleotides, sugars, nucleosides, organic acids, ketones, aldehydes, amines, amino acids, lipids, steroids, alkaloids, and small molecule drugs, are included in the study of metabolomics. The metabolite may arise from external sources, such as exposure to medications, toxins, or microbes, or it may be generated by the human host in the homeostatic process of energy utilization (**Fig. 1**). With growing interest in this field and improved

a Department of Cardiovascular Medicine, Heart & Vascular Institute, Cleveland Clinic, Cleveland, OH 44106, USA; b Department of Cardiovascular Medicine, Center for Clinical Genomics, Cleveland Clinic, Cleveland, OH 44106, USA
* Corresponding author. 9500 Euclid Avenue, Desk J3-4, Cleveland, OH 44195.
E-mail address: tangw@ccf.org

Heart Failure Clin 14 (2018) 109–118
http://dx.doi.org/10.1016/j.hfc.2017.08.011
1551-7136/18/© 2017 Elsevier Inc. All rights reserved.

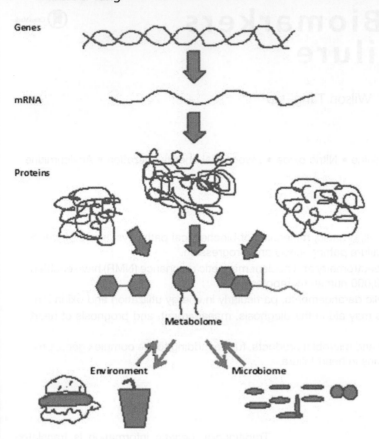

Genes

mRNA

Proteins

Metabolome

Environment   Microbiome

Fig. 1. Scheme of interactions of the metabolome with the genome, proteome, environment, and microbiome.

methods of identification, more than 40,000 unique metabolites have been identified in the Human Metabolome Database.[2] With this expansive list of metabolites, we are now poised with the opportunity to discover metabolomic biomarkers of the failing myocardium to facilitate in the early detection of heart failure,[3] appropriate targeted medical therapy of heart failure,[4] and offer prognostic insights into the progression of this disease. The study of metabolomics, then, represents another example of the spirit of translational research, bridging the gap from bench to bedside. This article will first examine the definition of a clinically useful biomarker, with respect to the biochemical utility of metabolomics, then delve into the methods of metabolomic profiling, examine several metabolomic pathways being pursued in heart failure (**Table 1**), present possible avenues of clinical application, and discuss challenges in the utilization of metabolomics.

METABOLITES AS BIOMARKERS: A PROLIFIC PROFILE

With advancements in technology, it is now feasible to generate large databanks of metabolites, and these extensive repositories of metabolites have become hypothesis generating in the pathogenesis

Table 1 Summary of metabolites in heart failure	
Metabolite	Findings in heart failure
Nitric oxide	Improves left ventricular dilation, vasodilation[14–16]
Arginine	Bioavailability and methylation affects nitric oxide synthesis[17–20]
Ketones	Myocardial metabolism switch from lipids to ketogenic state in heart failure[23,26]
Long-chain acylcarnitines	Myocardial metabolism switch in heart failure states[24,25]
Breath analysis of pentane, acetone, nitric oxide	Heart failure patients may expel a unique "breathprint"[28–31]
Trimethylamine N-oxide (host-gut microbiome interactions)	Elevated levels implicated in poor prognosis in myocardial infarction and chronic and acute heart failure[38,39,41–44,48]

of various diseases. For example, biochemical analysis of the human myocardium has revealed both its remarkable efficiency of energy utilization, as well as the pathologic alterations in biochemical substrate utilization in the failing myocardium.[5] As a metabolically active organ, the heart is in constant need for fuel, which comes in the form of adenosine triphosphate (ATP). Generation of ATP occurs either via catabolism, or breakdown, of exogenous molecules circulating in the blood, such as glucose, fatty acids, amino acids, or of endogenous stores of energy such as triacylglycerols or glycogen (**Fig. 2**).[6] In the healthy human heart, energy production occurs via efficient production of ATP with rapid turnover occurring every 10 seconds

such that the healthy heart metabolizes 30 g of fat and 20 g of carbohydrates daily.[7]

By understanding biochemical derangements occurring in heart failure, we can aim to produce metabolomic biomarkers as an indicator of presence of heart failure or gauge of the severity of cardiac metabolic dysregulation. Indeed, the concept of unique metabolomic patterns, or fingerprints, has already been validated in various small cohorts of patients with chronic heart failure.[8] The concept that unique patterns of metabolomic expression and energy utilization occur in different etiologies of heart failure could revolutionize the diagnosis and management of heart failure in this era of personalized medicine.

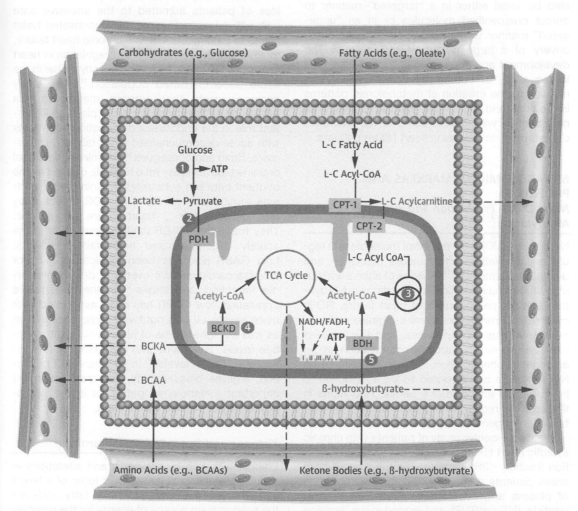

Fig. 2. Cellular metabolism and implications of metabolomic profiling. ATP, adenosine triphosphate; BCAA, branched-chain amino acid; BCKA, branched-chain α-keto-acid; BDH, β-hydroxybutyrate dehydrogenase; CoA, coenzyme A; CPT, carnitine palmitoyltransferase; FADH$_2$, flavin adenine dinucleotide; L-C, long-chain; NADH, nicotinamide adenine dinucleotide; PDH, pyruvate dehydrogenase; TCA, tricarboxylic acid. (*From* Ussher JR, Elmariah S, Gerszten RE, et al. The emerging role of metabolomics in the diagnosis and prognosis of cardiovascular disease. J Am Coll Cardiol 2016;68:2853; with permission.)

METABOLOMIC DISCOVERY

With the application of nuclear magnetic resonance (NMR) spectroscopy and mass spectrometry (MS), it is now feasible to efficiently analyze large volumes of metabolites derived from human samples, such as blood, urine, and gut contents. NMR allows for detection and quantification of metabolites based on chemical shifts in resonance frequency when subject to an electromagnetic field.[9,10] On the other hand, MS, identifies metabolites based on their unique mass/charge (m/z) ratio, and MS is often preceded by the use of gas chromatography, which separates metabolites based on solubility through a stationary media.[11,12] MS is more sensitive than NMR, and can detect a large quantity of metabolites. MS can also be used either in a "targeted" manner to detect prespecified molecules or in an "untargeted" manner without pre-specification for discovery of a large cohort of molecules.[13] The development and application of these techniques to the study of human myocardial metabolism has led to the creation of metabolomic patterns in healthy and pathologic cardiac states. The next section will address some of the examples of metabolomic studies in heart failure patients.

METABOLOMIC BIOMARKERS AND PROFILING
Nitric Oxide Production and Arginine Methylation

Nitric oxide (NO) is an important molecule that regulates vasodilation, left ventricular relaxation, and diastolic relaxation.[14–16] A series of animal and human studies have implicated alterations in NO synthesis in the pathogenesis of heart failure. NO is synthesized from its precursor L-arginine and oxygen by various NO synthases, and this process may be altered by arginine methylation in an epigenetic phenomenon. These alterations on NO synthesis are theorized to be a response to inflammation and oxidative stress. Alterations in the arginine regulation implicate its role in heart failure pathogenesis (**Fig. 3**).

In a single-center study of patients with chronic systolic heart failure with left ventricular (LV) ejection fraction $\leq$35%, plasma samples taken from these patients were analyzed for concentration of plasma aminoterminal pro-B-type natriuretic peptide (NT-proBNP) and endogenous arginine metabolites including asymmetric dimethylarginine (ADMA), symmetric dimethylarginine (SDMA), and N-mono-methylarginine (MMA).[17] ADMA inhibits nitric oxide synthase (NOS) activity, whereas SDMA does not. This study found

that both ADMA and SDMA plasma levels were positively correlated with echocardiographic estimates of LV filling pressures. In addition, the level of NT-proBNP was also correlated to all 3 arginine methylation products (MMA, ADMA, and SDMA), whereas no correlation was found with methyl-lysine, a metabolite with no NO inhibition, which was used as the internal control. Using Cox proportional hazard analysis, ADMA levels also increased the hazard ratio for death along, death or cardiac transplantation, and the combine endpoint of death, cardiac transplantation, or heart failure hospitalization. In addition, ADMA and MMA levels were lower in patients treated with beta-blocker, indicating response to therapy.

Another study compared the plasma metabolites of patients admitted to the intensive care unit with advanced, acute decompensated heart failure to patients with stable chronic heart failure, to elucidate the role of arginine regulation in heart failure. ADMA levels were significantly higher in the acute decompensated population.[18] This study again suggests that arginine metabolism via ADMA, an NO synthase inhibitor, plays an important role in the endothelial dysfunction in patients with acute decompensated heart failure. Furthermore, Shao and colleagues[18] examined the global arginine bioavailability ratio (GABR), defined as the quotient between substrates (arginine) and products (ornithine + citrulline) of NOS detected by MS, between the 2 heart failure populations. They found that GABR is significant lower in the acutely decompensated heart failure patients. Low GABR also has been implicated in major adverse cardiovascular events of death, myocardial infarction, and stroke.[19] In the heart failure population, low GABR has been associated with more severe LV and right ventricular dysfunction as well as higher levels of plasma natriuretic peptide levels. Treatment with beta-blocker therapy improves GABR levels.[20] In summary, NO regulation, arginine bioavailability, and methylation are important metabolomic pathways in the pathophysiology of cardiac dysfunction.

Ketones and Long-Chain Acylcarnitine

Energy utilization by the heart and alterations in cellular metabolism has been a topic of interest in heart failure research. Normally, fatty acids are the predominant source of energy for the myocardium. Acylcarnitines are the primary lipid substrate involved in fatty acid oxidation. Under normal metabolic conditions, β-oxidation produces 50% to 70% of ATP used by the myocardium.[21] Long-chain fatty acids, such as oleic and palmitic

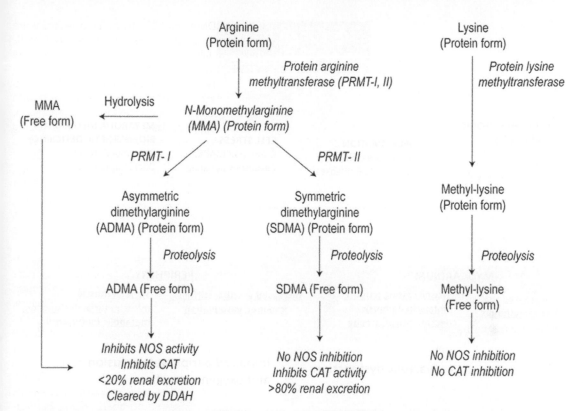

Fig. 3. Scheme of arginine metabolic pathways in high throughput MS arrays. ADMA, asymmetric dimethylarginine; CAT, cationic amino acid transport; DDAH, dimethylarginine dimethylaminohydrolase; MMA, N-mono-methylarginine; NOS, nitric oxide synthase isoforms; PRMT, protein arginine methyltransferases; SDMA, symmetric dimethylarginine. (*From* Tang WHW, Tong W, Shrestha K, et al..Differential effects of arginine methylation on diastolic dysfunction and disease progression in patients with chronic systolic heart failure. Eur Heart J 2008;29:2507; with permission.)

acids, are esterified into long-chain acylcarnitines (LCACs). LCACs then serve as lipid intermediates that transport carbon atoms into the mitochondrial for β-oxidation of fatty acids into triglycerides. In the failing myocardium, a metabolic switch from fatty acid utilization to oxygen-sparing carbohydrate metabolism has been observed.[22] This metabolic switch leads to accumulation of LCACs, which are postulated have pleotropic adverse effects on myocytes by way of promoting inflammation, increasing apoptotic signals, and generating ion channel dysregulation (**Fig. 4**).

Using liquid chromatography–MS in a nondiabetic advanced heart failure population of patients at time of heart transplantation or LV assist device implantation, Bedi and colleagues[23] evaluated the energy utilization in this group of patients with severe cardiac dysfunction. They found that failing myocardium increasingly used ketogenic β-hydroxybutyryl-CoA and β-hydroxybutyrate, while there was a decrease in the availability of lipid energetic substrates such as medium-chain and LCACs.

Other studies have assessed the metabolic derangements in heart failure with regard to energy utilization. In support of the metabolic switch theory by which the failing myocyte preferentially uses glucose rather than fatty acids, metabolic profiles of patients with chronic systolic heart failure reveal alterations in fatty acid metabolism. Ahmad and colleagues[24] evaluated a cohort of 453 patients with chronic systolic heart failure along with 41 end-stage heart failure patients undergoing left ventricular assist device (LVAD) implantation. Patients were randomized to exercise training versus usual care, and frozen plasma samples were collected and analyzed using MS. LCAC (C16 and C18) were associated with lower peak Vo_2 as well as increased risk of all-cause mortality, all-cause hospitalization, and cardiovascular death or hospitalization. Additionally, levels of long-chain acylcarnitine also decreased after placement of LVAD, suggesting response to therapy.

In a study that included both patients with heart failure with preserved ejection

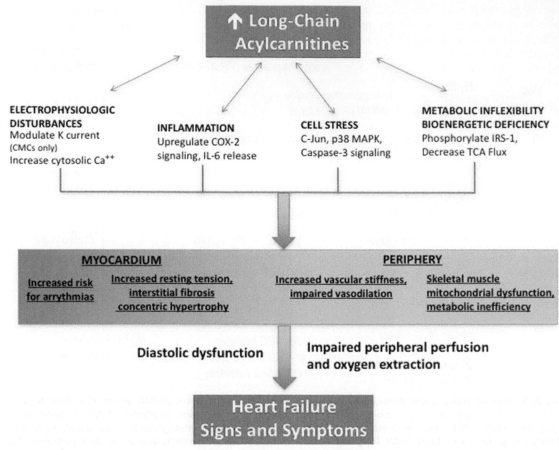

Fig. 4. Proposed model for plasma long-chain acylcarnitine contributions to the heart failure phenotype. Ca^{++}, calcium; CMC, cardiomyocyte; COX, cyclooxygenase; IL, interleukin; IRS, insulin receptor substrate; K, potassium; MAPK, mitogen-associated protein kinase; TCA, tricarboxylic acid. (*From* Hunter WG, Kelly JP, McGarrah RW 3rd, et al. Metabolomic profiling identifies novel circulating biomarkers of mitochondrial dysfunction differentially elevated in heart failure with preserved vs reduced ejection fraction: evidence for shared metabolic impairments in clinical heart failure. J Am Heart Assoc 2016;5(8):7; with permission.)

fraction ≥45% (HFpEF) and heart failure with reduced ejection fraction less than 45% (HFrEF), Hunter and colleagues[25] created metabolomic profiles of these patients to assess for differential alterations energy utilization. They quantified levels of 60 metabolites consisting of 45 acylcarnitines and 15 amino acids, expanding on an early study by Zordoky and colleagues.[8] These investigators find that elevated levels of LCAC were independently associated with worse functional status and higher mortality in both patients with HFpEF and HFrEF. Additionally, the level of LCAC was significantly higher in patients with HFrEF compared with HFpEF, and both heart failure phenotypes had elevated levels of LCAC compared with healthy controls. These studies further support the role of LCAC as a prognostic marker of disease severity in chronic systolic heart failure, as well as present potential

targets for new therapeutic interventions in heart failure.[26]

Human and Microbial Byproducts

Beyond analysis of plasma metabolites, the study of metabolomics also includes the analysis of human and microbial products and byproducts. A few tantalizing studies have evaluated the exhaled gases of patients with heart failure with respect to acetone, pentane, and other molecular excretion in the creation of a "breathprint" in chronic heart failure. The measurement of molecular concentrations via exhaled breath offers a major advantage in the noninvasive nature of the test, and several breath analysis test have already been approved by the Food and Drug Administration for the diagnosis of noncardiac conditions such as *Helicobacter pylori* infection, asthma inflammation, and carbon monoxide poisoning.[27] Within the cardiovascular realm, breath analysis studies have implicated that patients with heart failure have elevated levels of expired pentane, which is generated from the perioxidation reaction of free radicals with cellular membrane lipids.[28] In a similar manner, the concentration of exhaled acetone has also been implicated as a biomarker of heart failure severity.[29] Exhaled NO is another potential prognostic biomarker that has correlated to higher pulmonary venous hypertension in patients with stable chronic systolic heart failure.[30] Drawing from the previously mentioned studies, the feasibility of collecting exhaled breath samples in patients admitted with decompensated heart failure was validated in a recent proof of concept study.[31] Although breath analysis is subject to sampling discrepancy and requires careful collection methods, the analysis of exhaled breath gases and small molecules offers a noninvasive assessment of heart failure severity. A unique "breathprint" raises the possibility that unique metabolomic breath profiles can be used to identify and prognosticate patients with systolic heart failure.

Another area of interest has been intestinal flora metabolism in the pathogenesis of cardio-renal disease and heart failure. The intestinal microbiome is composed of trillions of commensal bacteria that populate gut and aid in digestion and absorption of nutrients. The interaction between microbacterial metabolism and different human disease states have recently been studied in the pathogenesis of insulin resistance, obesity, and cardiovascular disease.[32–37] Wang and colleagues[38] initially conducted hypothesis-generating studies to generate untargeted metabolomic maps to identify potential novel metabolites associated with cardiovascular risk. Through this work, 3 novel metabolites of the phosphatidylcholine (PC; lecithin) metabolism: choline (*m/z* 104), betaine (*m/z* 116), and trimethylamine N-oxide, TMAO, (*m/z* 76) were implicated in the pathogenesis of cardiovascular disease. Phosphatidylcholine is the major dietary source of choline in omnivores. Betaine is a direct oxidation product of choline, and TMAO is hypothesized to arise from bacterial metabolism of choline via the intermediate trimethylamine (TMA), and subsequent hepatic oxidation via flavin monooxygenase 3 (FMO3), forming TMAO. Of these 3 metabolites, TMAO demonstrated the strongest correlation to cardiovascular disease, which further implicates the role of the human and gut microbiome interactions that influence cardiovascular risk. TMAO has been linked to accelerated atherosclerosis and major adverse cardiac events (death, myocardial infarction, and stroke, **Fig. 5**).[39,40] TMAO also has been associated with poorer prognosis (death and myocardial infarction) at 2 years after myocardial infarction compared with GRACE (Global Registry of Acute Coronary Events) score or other biomarkers in coronary artery disease including

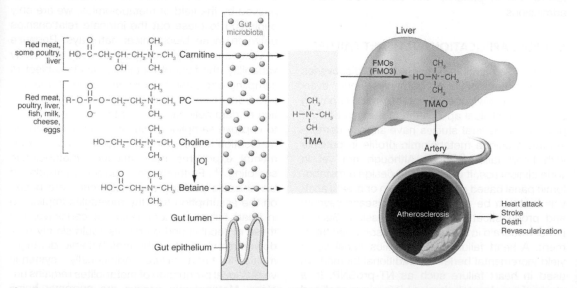

Fig. 5. Nutrient/meta-organismal pathway associated with atherosclerosis and major adverse cardiovascular events. FMO, flavin monooxygenase; O, oxidation; PC, phosphatidylcholine; TMA, trimethylamine; TMAO, trimethylamine *N*-oxide. (*From* Tang WHW, Hazen S. The contributory role of gut microbiota in cardiovascular disease. J Clin Investv 2014;124(10):4205; with permission.)

copeptin and natriuretic peptide, proenkephalin, mid-regional proadrenomedullin, and pro-substance P.[41]

In addition to atherosclerotic heart disease, elevated levels of TMAO have also been identified as a prognostic biomarker in patients with systolic heart failure. Mice fed high-choline diets have more severe pulmonary edema, cardiac enlargement, and LV ejection fraction.[42] In a large single-center study, Tang and colleagues[43] explored the incremental prognostic value of measuring TMAO levels in patients with stable chronic systolic heart failure. They found that TMAO correlates with BNP (R = 0.23; $P<.001$) and strong inverse correlation between TMAO and estimated glomerular filtration rate (eGFR, $r = -0.55$; $P<.001$). Furthermore, elevated TMAO levels portended higher long-term mortality that is independent of traditional biomarkers of risk in the heart failure population, such as BNP, eGFR, and markers of inflammation (hsCRP). Suzuki and colleagues[44] analyzed the predictive value of TMAO in patients admitted with acute decompensated heart failure. They found that the level of TMAO correlates with in-hospital mortality in patients admitted with acute heart failure when combined with clinical risk scores that include adjustment for renal function. Although the precise pathophysiologic contributions of TMAO in heart failure remain to be elucidated, the microbacterial-human gut metabolomic interaction presents a potential novel target for heart failure therapeutics both for chronic stable heart failure and in patients with acute heart failure admissions.

CLINICAL APPLICATIONS IN HEART FAILURE

With improvements in technology and discoveries in new metabolomics pathways, our ever-expanding knowledge of metabolomics is paving the way for clinical application in the heart failure population. Several studies have already demonstrated a unique metabolomic profile in patients with heart failure.[9,10,12,45] Although not yet in wide clinical use, it is feasible to design a metabolomic panel based on patient serum or breath analysis that can be used to gauge disease severity and prognosticate disease progression. Such a panel would aid in targeted and personalized treatment. A heart failure metabolomics panel could yield incremental benefit to traditional biomarkers used in heart failure such as NT-proBNP. In a study of novel metabolomics biomarkers analyzed by MS profiling, Cheng and colleagues[12] demonstrated that a metabolomic panel of novel biomarkers including histidine, phenylalanine,

spermidine, arginine, and phosphatidylcholine C34:4 have similar diagnostic value to BNP but have higher prognostic value for combined endpoints of death and heart failure–related hospitalization than BNP.

Metabolomic profiles can also be used to predict response to heart failure therapy. In small studies of patients undergoing ventricular assist device, trends in metabolomic biomarkers have indicated improvement in metabolomic profiles after LV unloading.[24] In patients undergoing cardiac resynchronization therapy (CRT), the assessment of metabolomic profiles have confirmed similar metabolomic derangements in patients with both ischemic and nonischemic systolic heart failure.[46] Although data appear controversial on baseline differences in metabolomic profiles between CRT-responders and CRT-nonresponders, some small prospective studies have indicated that CRT-responders have baseline differences in plasma concentrations of isoleucine, phenylalanine, leucine, glucose, valine, and glutamate.[47] This suggests that baseline metabolomic differences may be able to predict response to CRT and further prognosticate progression of heart failure in patients with severe LV dysfunction.

CHALLENGES AND POTENTIALS

Although advancements in technology have propelled the study of metabolomics in heart failure, many challenges and questions remain. Due to the diversity and complexity of molecular pathways and human-microbiome interactions encompassed by the field of metabolomics, we are only beginning to tease out the intricate relationships between these biochemical pathways. Because of vast variations in biological diversity and assay variability, the field of metabolomics is subject to sampling error, and the discrimination of true signals from noise remains challenging. Standardization of data collection methods would be needed to improve sampling accuracy, and alterations in medication history, dietary patterns, and environmental exposures may influence metabolomic sampling.[13] Furthermore, current methods of biomolecule profiling and discoveries are based on the assumption that the molecules implicated in heart failure pathogenesis are causative, but these molecules and pathways could simply be a downstream effect of the metabolomic derangements in heart failure. Additionally, systemic versus local production of metabolites remains unclear. Metabolomic assays are currently being used in other disease states such as mitochondrial diseases and inborn errors of metabolism; however, the analytical variability of samples, the instability of sample collection, and errors in collection have proved challenging in large-scale clinical use. Thus, the clinical application of metabolomics in heart failure remains limited at present time.

As the field of biomedical research has begun to discover the intricate biochemical pathways involved in disease pathogenesis, the field of medicine is moving toward more personalization of diagnostics, prognostics, and therapeutics. Metabolomics provides a more discrete dataset that is likely functionally impactful for human health and disease. Some studies have delved deeper into myocardial metabolism such as studies on ketone and acylcarnitines, whereas other discoveries, such as TMAO, have given us insights onto the host and microbial interactions that are implicated in heart failure pathogenesis. The study of small molecular compounds and pathways involved in heart failure represents an area of active clinical investigation. The creation of individualized metabolomic profiles in patients with heart failure could reveal novel pathways of heart failure pathogenesis, better define patients with a biochemical vulnerability for heart failure, and identify new targets of intervention. The study of metabolomics can also shed light onto the complex gene-environment interactions involved in heart failure onset and progression. We stand on the precipice of molecular discoveries that hold the potential to revolutionize the management of heart failure.

REFERENCES

1. Turer AT. Using metabolomics to assess myocardial metabolism and energetics in heart failure. J Mol Cell Cardiol 2013;55:12–8.
2. Wishart DS. HMDB 3.0—the human metabolome database in 2013. Nucleic Acids Res 2013;41: 801–7.
3. de Couto G, Ouzounian M, Liu PP. Early detection of myocardial dysfunction and heart failure. Nat Rev Cardiol 2010;7:334–44.
4. Griffin JL, Atherton H, Shockcor J, et al. Metabolomics as a tool for cardiac research. Nat Rev Cardiol 2011;8:630–43.
5. Kolwicz SC, Purohit S, Tian R. Cardiac metabolism and its interactions with contraction, growth, and survival of cardiomyocytes. Circ Res 2013;113: 603–16.
6. Ussher JR, Elmariah S, Gerszten RE, et al. The emerging role of metabolomics in the diagnosis and prognosis of cardiovascular disease. J Am Coll Cardiol 2016;68:2850–70.
7. Taegtmeyer H, Young ME, Lopaschuk GD, et al. Assessing cardiac metabolism: a scientific statement from the American Heart Association. Circ Res 2016;118:1659–701.
8. Zordoky BN, Sung MM, Ezekowitz J, et al. Metabolomic fingerprint of heart failure with preserved ejection fraction. PLoS One 2015;10:e0124844.
9. Deidda M, Piras C, Dessalvi CC, et al. Metabolomic approach to profile functional and metabolic changes in heart failure. J Transl Med 2015;13:297.
10. Tenori L, Hu X, Pantaleo P, et al. Metabolomic fingerprint of heart failure in humans: a nuclear magnetic resonance spectroscopy analysis. Int J Cardiol 2013;168:e113–5.
11. Senn T, Hazen SL, Tang WHW. Translating metabolomics to cardiovascular biomarkers. Prog Cardiovasc Dis 2012;55:70–6.
12. Cheng M-L, Wang CH, Shiao MS, et al. Metabolic disturbances identified in plasma are associated with outcomes in patients with heart failure: diagnostic and prognostic value of metabolomics. J Am Coll Cardiol 2015;65:1509–20.
13. Cheng S, Shah SH, Corwin EJ, et al. Potential impact and study considerations of metabolomics in cardiovascular health and disease: a scientific statement from the American Heart Association. Circ Cardiovasc Genet 2017;10:e000032.
14. Couto GK, Britto LRG, Mill JG, et al. Enhanced nitric oxide bioavailability in coronary arteries prevents the onset of heart failure in rats with myocardial infarction. J Mol Cell Cardiol 2015;86:110–20.
15. Azzam N, Zafrir B, Fares F, et al. Endothelial nitric oxide synthase polymorphism and prognosis in systolic heart failure patients. Nitric Oxide 2015;47:91–6.
16. Bhushan S, Kondo K, Polhemus DJ, et al. Nitrite therapy improves left ventricular function during heart failure via restoration of nitric oxide-mediated cytoprotective signaling. Circ Res 2014;114:1281–91.
17. Tang WHW, Tong W, Shrestha K, et al. Differential effects of arginine methylation on diastolic dysfunction and disease progression in patients with chronic systolic heart failure. Eur Heart J 2008;29:2506–13.
18. Shao Z, Wang Z, Shrestha K, et al. Pulmonary hypertension associated with advanced systolic heart failure: dysregulated arginine metabolism and importance of compensatory dimethylarginine dimethylaminohydrolase-1. J Am Coll Cardiol 2012;59: 1150–8.
19. Tang WHW, Wang Z, Cho L, et al. Diminished global arginine bioavailability and increased arginine catabolism as metabolic profile of increased cardiovascular risk. J Am Coll Cardiol 2009;53:2061–7.
20. Tang WWH, Shrestha K, Wang Z, et al. Diminished global arginine bioavailability as a metabolic defect in chronic systolic heart failure. J Card Fail 2013;19: 87–93.
21. Lopaschuk GD, Ussher JR, Folmes CDL, et al. Myocardial fatty acid metabolism in health and disease. Physiol Rev 2010;90:207–58.

22. Chokshi A, Drosatos K, Cheema FH, et al. Ventricular assist device implantation corrects myocardial lipotoxicity, reverses insulin resistance, and normalizes cardiac metabolism in patients with advanced heart failure. Circulation 2012;125:2844–53.

23. Bedi KC, Snyder NW, Brandimarto J, et al. Evidence for intramyocardial disruption of lipid metabolism and increased myocardial ketone utilization in advanced human heart failure. Circulation 2016; 133:706–16.

24. Ahmad T, Kelly JP, McGarrah RW, et al. Prognostic implications of long-chain acylcarnitines in heart failure and reversibility with mechanical circulatory support. J Am Coll Cardiol 2016;67:291–9.

25. Hunter WG, Kelly JP, McGarrah RW 3rd, et al. Metabolomic profiling identifies novel circulating biomarkers of mitochondrial dysfunction differentially elevated in heart failure with preserved versus reduced ejection fraction: evidence for shared metabolic impairments in clinical heart failure. J Am Heart Assoc 2016;5 [pii:e003190].

26. Kolwicz SC, Airhart S, Tian R. Ketones step to the plate: a game changer for metabolic remodeling in heart failure? Circulation 2016;133:689–91.

27. Cikach FS, Dweik RA. Cardiovascular biomarkers in exhaled breath. Prog Cardiovasc Dis 2012;55: 34–43.

28. Sobotka PA, Brottman MD, Weitz Z, et al. Elevated breath pentane in heart failure reduced by free radical scavenger. Free Radic Biol Med 1993;14: 643–7.

29. Marcondes-Braga FG, Gutz IGR, Batista GL, et al. Exhaled acetone as a new biomarker of heart failure severity. Chest 2012;142:457–66.

30. Schuster A, Thakur A, Wang Z, et al. Increased exhaled nitric oxide levels after exercise in patients with chronic systolic heart failure with pulmonary venous hypertension. J Card Fail 2012;18:799–803.

31. Samara MA, Tang WH, Cikach F Jr, et al. Single exhaled breath metabolomic analysis identifies unique breathprint in patients with acute decompensated heart failure. J Am Coll Cardiol 2013; 61:1463–4.

32. Dumas M-E, Barton RH, Toye A, et al. Metabolic profiling reveals a contribution of gut microbiota to fatty liver phenotype in insulin-resistant mice. Proc Natl Acad Sci U S A 2006;103:12511–6.

33. Dumas M-E, Kinross J, Nicholson JK. Metabolic phenotyping and systems biology approaches to understanding metabolic syndrome and fatty liver disease. Gastroenterology 2014;146:46–62.

34. Ridaura VK, Faith JJ, Rey FE, et al. Gut microbiota from twins discordant for obesity modulate metabolism in mice. Science 2013;341:1241214.

35. Turnbaugh PJ, Gordon JI. The core gut microbiome, energy balance and obesity. J Physiol 2009;587: 4153–8.

36. Turnbaugh PJ, Hamady M, Yatsunenko T, et al. A core gut microbiome in obese and lean twins. Nature 2009;457:480–4.

37. Turnbaugh PJ, Ley RE, Mahowald MA, et al. An obesity-associated gut microbiome with increased capacity for energy harvest. Nature 2006;444: 1027–31.

38. Wang Z, Klipfell E, Bennett BJ, et al. Gut flora metabolism of phosphatidylcholine promotes cardiovascular disease. Nature 2011;472:57–63.

39. Koeth RA, Wang Z, Levison BS, et al. Intestinal microbiota metabolism of L-carnitine, a nutrient in red meat, promotes atherosclerosis. Nat Med 2013;19: 576–85.

40. Tang WHW, Wang Z, Levison BS, et al. Intestinal microbial metabolism of phosphatidylcholine and cardiovascular risk. N Engl J Med 2013;368:1575–84.

41. Suzuki T, Heaney LM, Jones DJL, et al. Trimethylamine N-oxide and risk stratification after acute myocardial infarction. Clin Chem 2017;63:420–8.

42. Organ CL, Otsuka H, Bhushan S, et al. Choline diet and its gut microbe derived metabolite, trimethylamine N-oxide (TMAO), exacerbate pressure overload-induced heart failure. Circ Heart Fail 2016;9:e002314.

43. Tang WHW, Wang Z, Fan Y, et al. Prognostic value of elevated levels of intestinal microbe-generated metabolite trimethylamine-N-oxide in patients with heart failure: refining the gut hypothesis. J Am Coll Cardiol 2014;64:1908–14.

44. Suzuki T, Heaney LM, Bhandari SS, et al. Trimethylamine N-oxide and prognosis in acute heart failure. Heart 2016;102:841–8.

45. Du Z, Shen A, Huang Y, et al. 1H-NMR-based metabolic analysis of human serum reveals novel markers of myocardial energy expenditure in heart failure patients. PLoS One 2014;9:e88102.

46. Padeletti L, Modesti PA, Cartei S, et al. Metabolomic does not predict response to cardiac resynchronization therapy in patients with heart failure. J Cardiovasc Med (Hagerstown) 2014;15:295–300.

47. Nemutlu E, Zhang S, Xu YZ, et al. Cardiac resynchronization therapy induces adaptive metabolic transitions in the metabolomic profile of heart failure. J Card Fail 2015;21:460–9.

48. Tang WHW, Wang Z, Kennedy DJ, et al. Gut microbiota-dependent trimethylamine N-oxide (TMAO) pathway contributes to both development of renal insufficiency and mortality risk in chronic kidney disease. Circ Res 2015;116:448–55.

Printed and bound by CPI Group (UK) Ltd, Croydon, CR0 4YY

03/10/2024

01040382-0004